# Essential Practices in Hospice and Palliative Medicine

Fifth Edition

seems," said Grant.

Time was ticking away as the guys looked around for the probable location of a nearby phone.

"Guess we'll have to go find a police officer or someone that can help us, dang!" said Grant.

"No time, look, they're leaving!!" yelled August as he pounded his fists on the brick ledge in frustration.

With the van loaded up, two of the men jumped into the back, slamming the doors shut behind them. Shouting to his companions, Vasal ran around to the passenger side door and hopped in. The getaway driver, already in place, hit the gas, and the van peeled out now that all the men were on board.

The van's engine struggled and fought as the driver mashed down on the accelerator, pushing it to the floor. The sound of the museum alarm, ringing loudly in the thieves' ears, only heightened the sense of urgency in the driver as the thieves attempted to rapidly flee the scene. Lurching forward, the van sped right dead ahead toward where August and Grant stood.

Hustling, August and Grant dove out of the way just in the nick of time as the van screamed by them and took a sharp left turn down the hill.

"We've got to do something?!?!" yelled August looking around frantically for some answer!

"But what??!!!" roared Grant.

Spotting the bicycle across the street by the teenage boy, who by now had stopped reading and was looking up at all the commotion and noise coming from across the street, August, reacting more than thinking, ran over and grabbed the boy's bike, whirled it around and took off.

"Wait, whuh, huh, but that's my bike!!" croaked JJ from underneath the tree, while seeing his bicycle take off without him.

"I'm just borrowing it for a bit, I'll bring it right back, I promise!!" yelled August back to the boy behind him.

Peddling fast, August charged after the van as the bicycle clicked and rattled in protest, as he hurriedly changed gears.

"August, are you crazy, what do you think you're doing?!" bellowed Grant after his friend.

"Get to a phone, call the police, I'll try and keep up with them!" said August in hot pursuit.

At the bottom of the hill, going against traffic and swerving crazily, the van took an extremely sharp left turn, barely missing a direct collision with a pedestrian traffic light as it careened around in a wild circular arc toward the entrance to the bus tunnel. The skidding van burned rubber and painted dramatic tracks all over the road as it powered past the bus stop and into the tunnel.

Flying down the hill, August went sailing through the traffic light and intersection, making as sharp a turn as he possibly could without eating pavement, to chase after the van. With a near miss (or two!), he dodged oncoming traffic, causing motorists to slam on their brakes and skid to a stop as he charged past.

Up on the hill by the iron railing along the sidewalk, Grant tried desperately to call out to August before he disappeared from sight.

"August, wait!! August!!" he pleaded, waving his arms in exasperation.

But August couldn't hear him as he headed into the darkness of the tunnel, engulfed by uncertainty, hunting the van containing the stolen pieces of artwork, swallowed up in the chaos of the moment, his body surging with adrenaline-fueled strength.

Inside the dark underground bus tunnel, the sound of roaring engines echoed against the walls loudly. Chasing after the thieves, August biked as fast as he could to keep up with the van as it got further and further away in the scary chasm before him. The van driver had switched on the headlights, and in the dark August did his best to follow the taillights of the van as they grew ever fainter, like two eyes hiding in the night. With the light from the entrance fading and the incline of the road increasing, August began to struggle, as the depths of fatigue overtook him.

Up ahead the van's brake lights had come on strong, as the van was stuck behind a bus that had slowed to a crawl. Attempting to pass the cautious city bus, the van swerved wildly into the left lane, the driver realizing within nanoseconds that the reason the city bus had slowed was because another bus was coming from the other direction!! Wrenching the wheel hard to the right, the van's driver escaped colliding with the bus by less than a foot! August braced himself as best he could on the bicycle as the second bus barreled past him. In the distance, the faint light of the tunnel exit was growing larger and larger. The sweat poured off August as he forced himself to peddle. With the bus slowing the van down, August had nearly caught up with the thieves!

Rocketing out of the tunnel and past the slow city bus, August saw the van heading towards the busy intersection with Thayer Street straight ahead. The bright daylight was a bit disorienting to August and the thieves alike as they all tried to navigate life after the tunnel.

Inside the van, things were a bit tense! The driver was doing his best to stay on the road and keep their speed up, with the hope of getting lost in the crowd of car traffic exiting the city, to avoid police detection. Next to him, Vasal was barking orders.

"It's a one-way street! You can't turn left!!" yelled Vasal in the driver's ear, from the passenger seat.

Having passed the bus (which had now stopped completely at the tunnel exit, the bus driver not knowing at all what was going on) the thieves clung to their seats in the van as the bumpy ride continued. They had a choice to make regarding which route to take to help further their escape! Across from the tunnel exit there was a line of cars blocked by a bunch of pedestrians crossing the street.

"Quick, go right! Turn right!!!" shouted Vasal while pointing strongly and doing everything but grabbing the wheel himself.

Under pressure, he was starting to show signs of losing his cool. Heeding the high decibel directions reverberating off his eardrums, the driver radically coaxed the van to the right and made an abrupt 90-degree turn, clipping the edge of the sidewalk as they headed south on Thayer Street.

From twenty meters back, August saw that the van was turning right. Haphazardly, he weaved through the pedestrian traffic on the sidewalk, trying not to hit (or get hit!) as he bolted after the van. The chase had drawn a lot of attention, and turned heads all along Thayer Street as people stopped and stared at the unbelievable events that continued to unfold right before their eyes.

The 'Butternut Painting' van picked up speed as it hurtled down the street, with a handful of near misses of people and other obstacles. The gap between the van and August on the bike continued to widen as he pushed himself to keep up, his strength slowly giving out.

Looking through the dirty windshield and straight ahead, the thieves saw that up ahead on Thayer Street the traffic was moving at a snail's pace. Recognizing the danger of being slowed to a crawl, they had to make a lightning-quick decision.

"Argh, we can't be slowed down! Take this right, we'll head west and get onto the interstate, and put some distance between this city and us," ordered Vasal.

On cue, the driver took the recommended right turn as instructed. In the back, the other two thieves held the precious cargo steady and tried to lock themselves in position as the van leaned to the side around the curve. Their traumatized captives, the crooked painters, looked utterly terrified, and with the sharp turn of the van were flattened up against the side door and slammed into each other.

Recognizing up ahead that the van was turning yet again, August opted for a dramatic gamble in the hope of still catching up. Seeing to his right the large arched stone entranceway to the Brown University campus, he decided to try and cut across the school grounds and intercept the fleeing van. Pulse pounding, he swerved onto the sidewalk and raced through the archway.

On the other side, he followed the walkway at an angle, past the campus green where students were sitting studying, past the large equestrian statue of Marcus Aurelius he rode, racing between buildings, whizzing past students, and avoiding trees as he went.

In the distance, August heard the jarring sound of vehicles honking and could only assume that it was the getaway van. Over on George Street, heading west, the 'Butternut Painting' van containing the thieves had been forced to slow down, stuck behind an anxious driver who was completely befuddled by the tailgating van. The getaway driver kept blasting the van's horn over and over again and making the most awful racket, in an attempt at bullying the unfortunate car before them off the road.

Dashing across the college green, August made visual contact with the van in his left peripheral vision, making an adjustment on the fly for what would be an intercept course with the road. There was still a chance he could catch up with them! August was so close now, only ten meters from the street!

Meanwhile, spotting an opening in oncoming traffic, the driver of the van, fed up with being stuck behind the slow driver, made a brash move to pass. Accelerating forward, the engine of the van roared and growled as it blew past the slow driver.

Out the passenger's side window, an angry Vasal glowered at the pesky slow driver to vent his boiling frustration. At that moment, August reached the sidewalk and saw the van hurtling forward, but couldn't stop his bike in time…

Terror stricken, he tried to skid to a stop, but it was far too late, as his momentum carried him forward out into the street! Most onlookers covered their faces, unable to watch, while still others looked on in horror, trapped in a helpless gasp for air, unable to look away.

Flying out of control, August crashed right onto the street directly in the path of the speeding van as he panicked and the force of gravity took authority over the direction of the bicycle below him.

Completely caught off guard and with little time to react, the driver of the van slammed on the brakes and radically turned the wheel as hard to the left as his reflexes would allow.

Motion slowed. August could see the steel grill of the van rising in front of him. He closed his eyes with the hope that somehow the world would flinch first.

The rush of air was tremendous, as the van swerved to the left, tires squealing in protest, friction melting rubber, impact imminent. Heavy tires crushed the front of the bicycle into the asphalt, missing August's left leg by a thread.

Consequently, this drastic course alteration had put the van right in line to hit a parked navy blue mini-van. Colliding with the parked van, the thieves' vehicle practically did a full front flip as it twisted and turned in the air, mangling the parked vehicle in its path, before skidding to a stop down the street and resting on its side. In the distance, the sound of police sirens could be heard as people rushed to the aid of August and the occupants of the van.

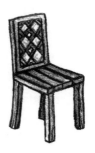

# CHAPTER FOURTEEN

In the corner of Headmaster Humboldt's Office, a vintage color TV set was tuned in to the local evening news. It was the six o'clock broadcast and the anchors were discussing that afternoon's breaking story out of the East Side of Providence!

"As you can see, police and rescue units were quick to respond to the accident here on George Street this afternoon, involving a van colliding with a second parked vehicle," droned on the news reporter.

Footage of the twisted wreckage flashed across the screen, the fierce red and blue glow of the lights of the many police and rescue vehicles giving the whole scene a very surreal look.

"Amazingly, no one was killed in the collision, as a driver and five passengers were involved in the crash. The police haven't confirmed whether or not there is a connection between this accident and the robbery at the art museum this afternoon. But we've been told by our sources that arrests are imminent," said the reporter.

"Additionally, we're hearing that the museum is reporting that nearly all of the art pieces taken from the museum today have been recovered and are unharmed."

Using a silver remote from his desk, Headmaster Humboldt clicked off the TV and swiveled his chair to face the two other people in the room.

Sitting in worn wooden chairs in front of the Headmaster's desk were August and Grant. A little shaken and with some bandages and wraps on August, the two were in surprisingly good shape, all things considered. Staring at both of them steadily, Headmaster Humboldt broke the silence.

"Anything else you'd like to tell me?" he asked gently.

Silence. The two boys were practically holding their breath, not knowing if they were about to get in trouble and endure the longest lecture of their lives or worse...

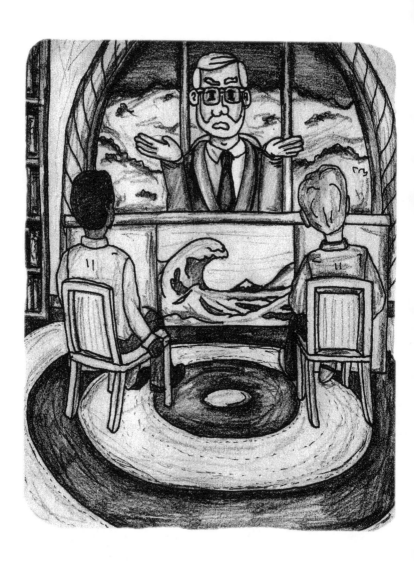

Taking off his glasses and cleaning them with a tissue, Headmaster Humboldt continued, all the while acting completely unfazed by the lack of a response to his opening line of questioning.

"No?" questioned Headmaster Humboldt, still directing his gaze at his captive audience.

Feeling brave, August decided to speak up.

"Well, there is one thing, sir. Well, it's more of a question really. Is Mr. Eastley okay? We were never able to reach him in the museum," asked August quietly.

With that, Headmaster Humboldt's gruff exterior broke down and a large smile spread across his face. Putting on his glasses, he slapped his own knee and chuckled loudly.

"Hah! Old Theodore? Yes, I spoke with him myself, he is fine, had quite a showdown with the art thieves apparently. But despite being knocked out with sleeping gas, he is no worse for the wear. He's as tough as they come, and I'm sure we're going to be hearing endlessly all about this latest tale of his, haha," laughed Headmaster Humboldt.

"That is a relief, sir. And the art thieves?" added Grant.

"Banged up pretty good from the collision, err, accident, and are currently in the hospital on close guard, but they'll all be fine. You did the right thing, Grant, reaching out to authorities so quickly. And how about you, August, how are you feeling? Put on quite a show, I hear!" said Headmaster Humboldt.

"I've felt better, sir, but nothing is broken. Except that poor boy's bike…" answered August.

"Yes, you'll have to arrange for the repairs to be made. I can recommend an excellent restorer of bicycles, does top-notch work," said Headmaster Humboldt.

"Who is it sir, do I know them?" asked August.

Pretending to look totally shocked and dismayed, Headmaster Humboldt jolted back in his chair.

"Why, me, of course!! Haven't you noticed what superb a shape my cycle is in?!" thundered Headmaster Humboldt.

"Oh, of course sir! That'd be wonderful, thank you sir!!" said August, feeling very relieved.

"Think nothing of it, you're welcome, and we'll make sure you have plenty of opportunities to give back to the community, in exchange, by taking care of some landscaping work here on the school grounds. Believe the maintenance director mentioned needing some extra help spreading mulch and raking leaves this coming week," said Headmaster Humboldt.

Unable to hide his dejection, August looked

rather defeated, and responded in kind.

"Right, looking forward to it sir," answered August glumly.

Knowing how August must feel, Grant couldn't help but interject into the conversation.

"Well, count me in too sir! I'll help August," exclaimed Grant.

Continuing to smile, Headmaster Humboldt looked quite pleased at the way everything was working out for the best.

"Very generous of you! I'm sure the director will be more than happy to have two helpers. Now I must say… that I am very proud of you both! The character and tenacity you fellows displayed under such trying conditions was most commendable," said Headmaster Humboldt, beaming.

"You really surprised me, congratulations to you both!" he added proudly.

Hearing praise coming from the headmaster, of all people, couldn't have shocked the boys more.

"Now, never, ever, ever, do it again! You both could have been killed!!! It was exceedingly reckless, not to mention monumentally foolish. Acting like a couple cowboys in the middle of the city, you both are very fortunate today! Now go outside, I believe there are a few people there waiting for you," said Headmaster Humboldt seriously, flipping gears once again.

Grins gone and jaws dropped by the impressive turnaround the headmaster had just pulled out of his proverbial hat; they gathered themselves to return to the dorms. Heading out the office door into the main hall of the administration building, they were met with a giant surprise!

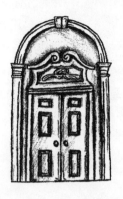

# CHAPTER FIFTEEN

The moment August and Grant stepped outside the headmaster's office and into the main hall of the administration building, with its vaulted ceilings and chandeliers, they were met with an enormous cheer!

Assembled in the hallway were dozens of students, including Winston, Shelby, Kasia, Penelope, Braylon, and Chloe, as well as other students they recognized from being in their classes and, of course, Mr. Eastley! There was resounding applause and all the faces were smiling back at them. August and Grant were stunned and overwhelmed by the response.

"You two make us all proud! Reminds me of the

time I rescued the nephew of the Maharaja and was later received in the palace as a guest of special honor," said Mr. Eastley, drawing loud, good-hearted applause, and chuckles of appreciation from those around him.

Continuing the revelry, another voice broke through the crowd.

"That's my little brother! And I taught him how to ride his first bike!" called out a proud Winston from the front lines.

Again, everyone cheered and August couldn't help but feel elated, knowing that his older brother was proud of him. Standing next to Winston, Grant and August saw Kasia and Penelope each holding up large neon signs. In blinding, bold colors the first sign read 'You guys totally bailed on us this afternoon!!' with the second saying 'But we forgive you!!'

"And we want a rain check, okay?" shouted Kasia, not able to wait a moment longer.

"Well, what do you say??!" she demanded.

Laughing at the zaniness of the proceedings, both August and Grant (who was slightly blushing) nodded in reply. This caused more applause and carrying on from the crowd. Yet, faintly, those who listened closely would hear a small voice trying to make itself heard above the din of all the cheering and clapping.

"I know them! I know them! They're my neighbors, next-door!!" peeped Shelby from the back. With that the crowd cheered the loudest yet!

Walking up next to August and Grant, by his open office door, Headmaster Humboldt addressed the crowd.

"Thank you, yes, thank you to everyone for coming tonight to honor the achievements of these fine young men, who model the noble spirit that is within us all. For it is when challenges arise that true character is shown. And standing here, I am reminded by their actions and their friendship that we should all strive to share the very best of ourselves. And let the difficulties of our lives and our times reveal the courage, goodness, and strength within," said Headmaster Humboldt.

Thoughtfully listening to the headmaster's words, the crowd had gone very quiet, as they took it all in and gave him their full attention.

"Now I think it is time to let our heroes get some rest, as they've had a very full day," added Headmaster Humboldt.

Once more, everyone applauded, and Headmaster Humboldt returned to his office, while August and Grant ventured out into the hall surrounded by all their friends.

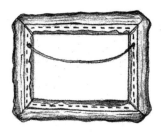

# CHAPTER SIXTEEN

[SEVERAL DAYS LATER]

Wednesday night had arrived, and August, Grant, and Shelby were hanging out in the guys' dorm room. All the excitement from the events of the past weekend had died down, and things were starting to return to normal again. Shelby was sitting at August's desk going over some schematics for his latest invention and thinking quietly to himself. Grant was scrounging around by the TV, trying to finally get the videogame systems set up so that they could actually play them.

"Alright guys, I think I got it this time! All the

cables check out and I've reworked the flow of power bars, so we should definitely be in business!" Grant said confidently, while plugging in the last AC adapter.

Sitting on his bed, August was engrossed reading the newspaper and paying close attention to the cover article on the robbery.

"It says here that authorities have recovered all but one of the paintings stolen from the art museum on Saturday. Four arrests have been made in the case, but Titian's masterwork 'The Venus of Urbino' seems to have disappeared without a trace," said August.

Finished reading, he laid down the newspaper on the patchwork quilt covering his bed.

"Can't believe they still haven't found it yet, where could it be??" wondered August aloud.

"Clearly the investigators are missing something. A painting doesn't just get up and walk off by itself," said Shelby.

"I don't know anything about that, but what I do know is no one here can stop me in this game. Anyone willing to try?" boasted Grant.

Holding out a game controller to anyone who dared challenge him, he was prepared to take on all comers.

"You remember what happened last time you

fired that thing up?" chuckled August, half serious, half joking.

"Oh, not to worry, it's all fixed now, I swear!" declared Grant, doing everything but patting himself on the back in congratulations.

Taking the controller from him, August sat down to play a head-to-head match-up against Grant in his favorite classic videogame. Shelby watched with mild curiosity from the desk as Grant prepared to turn on the system.

"No way it doesn't work this time!" he said confidently.

Pressing the 'on' switch, the videogame system powered up straight away, which August took as a very good sign! Now Grant turned on the TV. Everything was working, so far so good! Very proudly, Grant marveled over his own technological achievement in getting it to cooperate for him this time around.

"See, I told you. No problem at all," he said.

Blip. Just like that, all the power went out and the room was draped in pure darkness.

"Nooooooo!!!! Not again!!!" croaked Grant.

Unable to hold in their laughter for even a second, Shelby and August broke and couldn't contain themselves. Unable to see much of anything in front of him, Grant frantically pressed buttons and tried to get anything to happen.

"I don't believe this! I seriously can't believe this is happening again!" he yelled.

Everything was totally dark, and the sound of Grant's frustration and aggravation over the repeat of the blown fuse was taking center stage.

"I fixed it! That totally should have worked!" grumbled Grant. "Stop laughing you guys. I really did this time; I re-configured the whole blasted thing! This is ridiculous! What am I going to do now?!" he yelled.

Flying twenty-thousand feet overhead, the sound of a jet plane can faintly be heard over the boys' laughter. Bright moonlight was reflecting off the hull of the plane as it rose up through the cover of the nighttime clouds to reach the peaceful realm above under the starry sky. Inside the cabin of the small, private, chartered jet plane were incredible plush leather reclining seats. Everything about this plane screamed luxury and made any passenger feel like royalty.

Tonight, these glamorous accommodations were reserved for a singularly such fortunate passenger. Sitting very comfortably in one of the exquisite seats was a woman wearing all black. She was holding a travel book about Tuscany and flipping through its pages.

Resting beside her, wrapped up in canvas and twine was a rectangular object that looked to be about four feet tall by five and a half feet wide in size.

A flight attendant approached the woman with a tray of drinks.

"Would you like another coffee, or a cappuccino, perhaps?" she asked politely.

"No, thank you. I have everything I need!" replied Lexi. Smiling, she returned to her reading, all the while quietly keeping a very close eye on her canvas-wrapped traveling companion, glancing at it every once in awhile, as if still in awe at its very presence.

THE END

Made in the USA
Middletown, DE
22 January 2015

# Essential Practices in Hospice and Palliative Medicine
Fifth Edition

## UNIPAC 9
# HIV, DEMENTIA, AND NEUROLOGICAL CONDITIONS

**Christopher M. Blais, MD MPH FAAHPM**
Ochsner Health System
Ochsner Medical Center
New Orleans, LA

**Jennifer Gabbard, MD**
Wake Forest Baptist Health
Wake Forest School of Medicine
Winston-Salem, NC

**Sonia Malhotra, MD MS FAAP**
University Medical Center
Tulane University School of Medicine
Louisiana State University School of
  Medicine
New Orleans, LA

**Susan E. Nelson, MD FACP FAAHPM**
Franciscan Missionaries of Our Lady Health
  System
Baton Rouge, LA

*Reviewed by*
**Matthew T. Mendlik, MD PhD**
University of Pennsylvania
Philadelphia, PA

*Edited by*
**Joseph W. Shega, MD**
Vitas Healthcare
Miami, FL

**Miguel A. Paniagua, MD FACP**
University of Pennsylvania
Philadelphia, PA

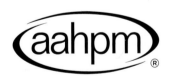

AMERICAN ACADEMY OF
HOSPICE AND PALLIATIVE MEDICINE

8735 W. Higgins Rd., Ste. 300
Chicago, IL 60631
aahpm.org | PalliativeDoctors.org

The information presented and opinions expressed herein are those of the editors and authors and do not necessarily represent the views of the American Academy of Hospice and Palliative Medicine. Any recommendations made by the editors and authors must be weighed against the healthcare provider's own clinical judgment, based on but not limited to such factors as the patient's condition, benefits versus risks of suggested treatment, and comparison with recommendations of pharmaceutical compendia and other medical and palliative care authorities.

Some discussions of pharmacological treatments in *Essential Practices in Hospice and Palliative Medicine* may describe off-label uses of drugs commonly used by hospice and palliative medicine providers. "Good medical practice and the best interests of the patient require that physicians use legally available drugs, biologics, and devices according to their best knowledge and judgment. If physicians use a product for an indication not in the approved labeling, they have the responsibility to be well informed about the product, to base its use on firm scientific rationale and on sound medical evidence, and to maintain records of the product's use and effects. Use of a marketed product in this manner *when the intent is the 'practice of medicine'* does not require the submission of an Investigational New Drug Application (IND), Investigational Device Exemption (IDE), or review by an Institutional Review Board (IRB). However, the institution at which the product will be used may, under its own authority, require IRB review or other institutional oversight" (US Food and Drug Administration, https://www.fda.gov/RegulatoryInformation/Guidances/ucm126486.htm. Updated January 25, 2016. Accessed May 17, 2017.).

Published in the United States by the American Academy of Hospice and Palliative Medicine, 8735 W. Higgins Rd., Ste. 300, Chicago, IL 60631.

**AAHPM Education Staff**
Julie Bruno, Director, Education and Learning
Angie Forbes, Manager, Education and Learning
Kemi Ani, Manager, Education and Learning
Angie Tryfonopoulos, Coordinator, Education and
  Learning

**AAHPM Editorial Staff**
Jerrod Liveoak, Senior Editorial Manager
Bryan O'Donnell, Managing Editor
Andie Bernard, Assistant Editor
Tim Utesch, Graphic Designer
Jean Iversen, Copy Editor

ISBN 978-1-889296-29-6

# Contents

# Tables

# Figures

# Acknowledgments

AAHPM is deeply grateful to all who have participated in the development of this component of the *Essential Practices in Hospice and Palliative Medicine* self-study program. The expertise of the editors, contributors, and reviewers involved in the current and previous editions of the *Essentials* series has ensured the value of its content to our field.

AAHPM extends special thanks to the authors of previous editions of this content: Vincent Jay Vanston, MD FAAHPM, Shubhra M. Shetty, MD FACP, Carla S. Alexander, MD, Gary S. Reiter, MD, Joseph W. Shega, MD, and Stacie K. Levine, MD; the pharmacist reviewer for this edition of the *Essentials* series, Jennifer Pruskowski, PharmD; the authors of the *UNIPAC 9 amplifire* online learning module, Jennifer Gabbard, MD, Sonia Malhotra, MD, and Susan E. Nelson, MD FACP FAAHPM; and the many professionals who volunteered their time and expertise to review the content and test this program in the field—Joseph Rotella, MD MBA HMDC FAAHPM, Jonathan S. Appelbaum, MD, Anthony Back, MD, Dominic F. Glorioso, DO, Robert Hirschtick, MD, Carol F. Knight, EdM, Harlee Kutzen, MN ACRN, Sharon Lee, MD, Stacie K. Levine, MD, Kathleen McGrady, MD MS MA FAAHPM, Frederick J. Meyers, MD, Steven Oppenheim, MD, James B. Ray, PharmD, Pamela Sass, MD, Joseph W. Shega, MD, C. Porter Storey, Jr., MD FACP FAAHPM, Malgorzata Sullivan, MD, Jay Thomas, MD PhD, and Charles von Gunten, MD PhD FACP.

*Essential Practices in Hospice and Palliative Medicine* was originally published in 1998 in six volumes as the *UNIPAC* self-study program. The first four editions of this series, which saw the addition of three new volumes, were created under the leadership of C. Porter Storey, Jr., MD FACP FAAHPM, who served as author and editor. AAHPM is proud to acknowledge Dr. Storey's commitment to and leadership of this expansive and critical resource. The Academy's gratitude for his innumerable contributions cannot be overstated.

## Continuing Medical Education

Continuing medical education credits are available, and Maintenance of Certification credits may be available, to users who complete the *amplifire* online learning module that has been created for each volume of *Essential Practices in Hospice and Palliative Medicine*, available for purchase from aahpm.org.

—

# HIV/AIDS

## History and Development of HIV/AIDS

### Facts and Figures

First reported in 1981, acquired immunodeficiency syndrome (AIDS) quickly became a leading cause of death for young adults in the United States. In the early 1980s the human immunodeficiency virus (HIV) epidemic was concentrated in homosexual Caucasian males. By the late 1980s injection drug use emerged as a major mode of HIV transmission. From this population, the disease then quickly spread to heterosexual and pediatric populations. In the first 14 years, sharp increases in the number of new AIDS diagnoses and deaths among people 13 years and older were reported, reaching highs of 75,457 in 1992 and 50,628 in 1995, respectively. With the introduction of highly active antiretroviral therapy (ART), AIDS diagnoses and deaths declined substantially from 1995 to 1998 and remained stable from 1999 to 2008, with an average of 38,279 AIDS diagnoses and 17,489 deaths per year. Despite the decline in AIDS cases and deaths, by 2015 an estimated 1.1 million people in the United States were living with HIV, and 14% of these people had undiagnosed infection.[1,2]

The challenges in the developed world differ significantly from those in the developing world. Despite better access to diagnosis and treatment in the developed world, relatively late diagnosis, adherence issues, and emerging resistance to drugs are ongoing issues. Although public attitudes toward people living with AIDS have improved, fear and stigma are still major impediments to seeking and continuing care.

In the United States HIV disproportionately affects people of color and those with low socioeconomic status. In 2015 an estimated 69% of individuals newly diagnosed with HIV/AIDS were Hispanic/Latino or African American. At every stage, from HIV diagnosis until death, the racial or ethnic group affected the most is African Americans. Although African Americans account for only 12% of the US population, they represent almost half of the estimated number of diagnosed HIV/AIDS cases.[2]

Treatment for HIV/AIDS has changed dramatically since the mid 1990s. Before the arrival of protease inhibitors (PIs) and highly active ART, a diagnosis of AIDS predicted a mean survival of approximately 1 year. The arrival of PIs in 1996 resulted in dramatic decreases in HIV-related mortality in the industrialized world, with declines in death rates of 50% to 60% in the United States and Europe between 1996 and 2000.[3] ART transformed HIV/AIDS into a manageable chronic disease. From 2010 through 2014, the annual estimated number and rate of diagnoses of HIV infection in the United States remained stable.[4]

### Challenges

The advent of ART and the transformation of HIV/AIDS into a chronic disease have resulted in new and growing challenges. For example, although there is an overall decrease in AIDS deaths, there has been no change in the incidence of new HIV infections. The combination of these two factors has resulted in an increased number of people living with symptomatic HIV disease for longer periods.

In fact, the life expectancy of patients with HIV has improved markedly. The potential ambulatory care of these patients now spans several decades, underscoring the importance of continuity, longitudinal care, and awareness of aging-related issues. Approximately 75% of the population living with HIV in the United States is 40 years or older. Worsening immune function, multiple comorbidities, socioeconomic stressors, financial strain, and isolation all may lead to early frailty, disability, and mortality in this population.[5]

Coincident with improved survival, the patterns of morbidity and mortality have changed among patients who are HIV-positive. Cardiovascular disease, hypertension, and diabetes have become prevalent. With prolonged survival, causes of death have shifted from opportunistic infections to end-stage liver disease, end-stage kidney disease, and non-HIV-related malignancies.[3,6,7]

From a public health perspective, issues of inequality and justice persist for people with HIV. Poorer communities have higher rates of HIV/AIDS, and patients with low socioeconomic status have higher morbidity and mortality.[8-11] Inadequate insurance, unstable housing, mental illness, and substance abuse all lead to inconsistent care and poor outcomes. From a global perspective, with stark differences in quality of and access to care between developed and developing countries, huge disparities exist.[12,13]

Despite advances in treatment, no cure has been found for HIV infection. It remains a lifelong disease that requires constant monitoring and treatment. The complexity of HIV treatment, the rising incidence of complex comorbidities, and the persistence of marked psychosocial and spiritual issues underscore the importance of concurrent palliative care throughout the course of this disease. As the medical treatment of HIV/AIDS becomes increasingly complex, the tendency to "medicalize" treatment regimens also increases, with less attention given to the psychosocial and spiritual needs of patients and their families. It is critical that palliative care providers overcome this tendency and develop close working relationships with all healthcare providers.

## Clinical Situation

### Rajesh

Rajesh is referred to your hospice program with a diagnosis of end-stage AIDS. The referring physician is an internist who has cared for Rajesh and his family for years. Rajesh is married to a man and has three children from a previous marriage, all of whom are in college. He is a software developer for a local computer company and travels frequently.

Twelve months ago Rajesh developed fevers, night sweats, and weight loss. His internist has seen him frequently and evaluated him extensively for cancer, collagen vascular disease, and tropical diseases. Upon finding thrush in Rajesh's oropharynx, he suggests an HIV test. The test came back positive. Subsequent HIV viral load and CD4 counts were 150,000 copies/cc and 35 cells/mcL, respectively. His complete blood count (CBC) shows white-blood-cell (WBC) count 1.2 (40 segs, 4 bands, 21 lymphs, 19 monos, 5 eos, and 11 basos), Hgb 9 g, and platelet count 77; chemistries show albumin 1.8 g/dL and total protein 8.5 g/dL; liver function tests are normal.

On examination you find that Rajesh is 5-ft 11-in tall and weighs 140 lb (normal adult weight for him is 180 lb). He has oropharyngeal thrush; his fundi are clear. He has cervical, axillary, and inguinal adenopathy. His liver and spleen are not enlarged. His genitals are normal. His rectal examination shows plaque-like white lesions in the perianal area.

You speak with Rajesh and discover that he has been engaging in unsafe sex with men when he is traveling for his job. He is shocked about his diagnosis and is terrified to tell his husband and children. He is having trouble sleeping and eating and is no longer interested in his old hobbies or work.

 What is the most appropriate next step at this point?

*Case continues on page 9*

## Quality of Life

The overall goal of palliative care is to improve patients' quality of life (QOL) by relieving or reducing suffering.[14] Despite increasingly prolonged survival times, patients with HIV continue to experience physical and spiritual distress, psychological pain, social isolation, and grief.[15] Healthcare professionals must carefully assess for pain, fatigue, depression, spiritual distress, anorexia, and other symptoms that may be present even when disease markers are improving.[16] Clinicians also must anticipate therapy-related side effects and be prepared to offer effective interventions for preventing or controlling them.

The best guide for providing effective care is the patient's responses to questions about current QOL and important goals. Traditionally, scales for measuring QOL primarily have reflected functional status. Scales designed to elicit information about symptoms, including psychological and spiritual distress, are more likely to be helpful (see *UNIPAC 2*).

Patients with HIV infection frequently have more than one active problem. Prioritizing problems and discussing each separately can be very useful for patients, caregivers, and clinicians. This is especially true for patients with underlying psychiatric conditions, a common occurrence for patients with a history of intravenous (IV) drug use.

Continuing to address psychosocial and spiritual concerns for patients with advanced HIV infection is important. When a person is healthy, the thought of being bedridden might seem unbearable. However, as death approaches, priorities often shift. Relationships, spiritual issues, and taking pleasure in the moment often become more important. When comprehensive palliative care is provided, including interventions to alleviate psychological and spiritual suffering, it is not unusual for people to rate their QOL as higher during this period because they can focus on achieving personal goals rather than accomplishing the usual, mundane tasks of life (see *UNIPAC 2*). **Table 1** lists some of the common QOL issues related to HIV/AIDS.

Finding effective interventions to improve the QOL of individuals living with HIV/AIDS remains a challenge. Numerous programs continue to be developed and tested. Support through peer-based interventions and early case management shows promise.[17,18]

A number of studies have focused specifically on the QOL of women with HIV.[19,20] These studies have consistently found that social factors and psychological symptoms have a major impact on a woman's QOL.[21-26] Women reporting HIV discrimination had higher mean scores for stress, suicidal ideation, depressive symptoms, and number of unprotected sexual episodes. They were also found to have lower mean scores for self-esteem and QOL.[27,28]

The same activities that put women at risk for HIV also put them at risk for significant psychosocial distress. In one study of both HIV-positive women and HIV-negative women at high risk for infection, the rates of significant depressive symptoms and adverse life events exceeded 60%.[29,30] These adverse life events included[31]

- a high prevalence of physical abuse and childhood sexual abuse
- domestic violence
- substance abuse
- inadequate family or social support
- sex trading.

Such factors clearly have a negative impact not only on QOL but also on adherence with treatment and mortality. These findings strongly emphasize the importance of comprehensive screening as well as early psychosocial support and intervention.

As with other chronic diseases, those suffering from substance abuse and psychiatric disorders remain particularly vulnerable. Studies consistently show that patients infected with HIV with untreated psychiatric and substance abuse problems have a lower QOL and suffer higher morbidity and mortality compared with those infected with HIV alone.[32]

## Prognosis

Assessing prognosis and risk of progression to end-stage AIDS and death is guided by multiple factors, including a patient's response to ART, AIDS-associated conditions, and personal behaviors. None of these factors alone can predict disease progression. Instead, the best guides

## Table 1. Common Quality of Life Issues Related to HIV/AIDS

Physical symptoms related to HIV infection and treatment

Partners, spouses, and caregivers who are HIV-positive with their own illness-related symptoms and death-related fears

Unpredictable course of disease and attendant chronic emotional distress

Denial of disease progression on the part of dying patients, caregivers, and physicians

Social isolation related to the stigma associated with HIV infection

HIV-related dementia and related concerns (eg, appointing a healthcare proxy)

Psychiatric problems such as anxiety, depression, and schizophrenia

Substance abuse

Spiritual issues related to the stigma associated with HIV infection and premature disability and death

Poverty-related issues, including inadequate funds for expensive medications, home care, and supplies

Limited access to experienced healthcare professionals in rural areas

Ability of grandparents to care for grandchildren whose parents have died from AIDS

for gauging prognosis are careful assessments of all contributing factors and consultations with a physician experienced in treating individuals with HIV infection.

### Assessment of Prognosis

Without treatment, the duration of AIDS development is highly variable, ranging from 2 to 3 years to no signs of AIDS development in the patient's entire lifetime. The rate of AIDS progression is divided into three major types:

- slow progression, during which AIDS develops slowly between a span of 3 to 10 years after seroconversion
- long-term nonprogression, during which an undetectable or low level of HIV ribonucleic acid (RNA) is present for more than 10 years
- rapid progression, during which AIDS develops within 3 years of seroconversion.

Disease progression for individuals with HIV depends on a combination of viral, host, and environmental factors.[33]

In the early phase of the epidemic, mortality was readily and uniformly predicted by the occurrence of specific opportunistic infections and surrogate markers like the CD4 count and the HIV viral load. Before the introduction of ART, median survival for people with a CD4 count below 50 cells/mcL ranged between 12 and 27 months. With CD4 counts less than 20 cells/mcL, median survival dropped to 11 months. Conditions suggestive of a survival of 6 months or less were developed by the National Hospice Organization in 1996.[34] These ranges may be applicable to contemporary patients not on ART because of lack of access to care, side effects, compliance problems, or multidrug resistance.[35] Today these prognostic markers are much less reliable in late-stage disease, and virtually any of the traditional prognostic markers may be overridden by the potential impact of ART.[36] For example, because of the success of ART since 1996 as well as improvements in the prevention and treatment of HIV complications, more than 80% of patients are now alive 10 years after seroconversion. In addition, patients with CD4 counts higher than 200 cells/mcL are more likely to die from an illness unrelated to HIV than they are from complications of AIDS.[35,37]

As deaths from opportunistic infections have declined, mortality from other comorbidities has become more common (eg, hepatitis B and C infection, renal failure, non-HIV-related cancers, cardiovascular disease, suicide, complications from substance abuse).[38,39]

The Antiretroviral Therapy Cohort Collaborative, which includes 19 cohort studies from Europe and North America, was established to estimate prognosis for patients who had HIV-1 infection and were treatment naive when initiating ART. Factors considered include age, CD4 count, viral load, US Centers for Disease Control and Prevention (CDC) classification stage, and HIV transmission through IV drug use. Risk calculators[40] produce estimates for progression rates at years 1 to 5 after the initiation of ART.[41]

When assessing prognosis, hospice professionals and HIV clinicians should consider the patient's response to therapy, any comorbid conditions, the patient's wishes, and any of the patient's personal behaviors that may increase the risk of disease progression. In general, a patient on ART with an elevated HIV viral load, a depressed and dropping CD4 cell count (fewer than 50 cells/mcL),[42] multidrug-resistant HIV, cachexia, and objective clinical deterioration has a very poor prognosis. Other associated comorbidities and behaviors worsen the prognosis. One study suggests that functional deficits or the existence of other life-threatening conditions (eg, cancer, end-organ failure) predict short-term mortality for patients with advanced HIV disease.[36] See **Table 2** for a list of common comorbid illnesses that predict poor outcomes or death for people with HIV.

No patient with AIDS should be given a terminal prognosis until a physician with expertise in the treatment of patients with HIV has completed a thorough evaluation of the patient's condition. Many patients who appear quite ill can improve dramatically and resume a normal life when treated with state-of-the-art ART and appropriate opportunistic disease prophylaxis or treatment, as indicated.

### Behaviors that Increase Risk of Disease Progression

Intractable substance abuse increases the risk of disease progression and the development of life-threatening comorbid illnesses. Incomplete adherence to antiretroviral medications, the primary cause of antiretroviral failure, is associated with substance abuse.[44,46] Incomplete adherence also predisposes individuals to the development of viral resistance and subsequent disease progression. Alcohol abuse accelerates the progression of chronic viral hepatitis and predisposes patients to malnutrition, which worsens prognosis.

Social isolation, a general lack of social support, and stigma associated with HIV disease are also associated with worsened prognosis. Poor medication adherence is more common with

## Table 2. Comorbid Illnesses Predicting Poor Outcomes in People with HIV[36,43-45]

Hepatic decompensation (often related to hepatitis C cirrhosis)

Non-Hodgkin lymphoma, if unresponsive to therapy

Hodgkin lymphoma, if unresponsive to therapy

Progressive multifocal leukoencephalopathy

Primary central nervous system lymphoma

Diarrhea for longer than 1 month

Low body mass index

Any metastatic neoplasm

Intractable substance abuse

Psychiatric illness, if unresponsive to therapy

Any opportunistic infection unresponsive to therapy

socially isolated individuals, who may lose the will to fight a treatable but demanding chronic illness like HIV infection.[47-51] In one study of adolescents and young adults with HIV who presented at a public primary care facility, participants described the challenges of adhering to medications when in the presence of friends, families, doctors, and even themselves, from whom they wished to hide or deny their status.[52]

## *Realistic Goal Setting and Advance Care Planning*
### Maintaining Hope

To provide the most supportive and sensitive care throughout a patient's illness, healthcare professionals must periodically reassess the patient's goals. Just as QOL evolves, so do desired outcomes. Although many healthcare professionals fear that discussions about realistic, achievable goals and desired outcomes may take away a patient's hope, this is not the case.[53,54] Most patients, partners, and family members appreciate compassionate, truthful discussions of the patient's prognosis and want to be included in decision making because it enhances their sense of control over a distressing situation.

Patients report that a sense of hope helps sustain them through difficulties. Supporting hope does not mean supporting false expectations; instead, it encourages patients to redefine hope as their illness progresses. When hope for a long life is no longer sustainable, patients may hope for meaningful days or for the chance to leave lasting memories for friends or family members by making a scrapbook, an audiotape, or a video.[55] Multiple studies document that a sense of spiritual well-being positively affects a patient's QOL (see *UNIPAC 2*).

### Personal Goals

All people have goals and wishes, some of which are unacknowledged and unspoken. Members of the care team should help patients identify their goals and determine how they might be realized, if only in part. When discussing goals, care providers will find it useful to gently ask patients questions such as "What aspects of your life are most important to you?" and "What in your life makes you feel proud?" Patients frequently report that important goals include participating in a family anniversary or living long enough to see an expected grandchild. Patients may want to spend time identifying the people they care about most and those who will serve as their primary base of support as their condition deteriorates.

Young patients with HIV infection may not have had time to realize any of their dreams. In such cases, the team must acknowledge the pain of unachieved dreams, help patients value the lives they have lived, and help them identify ways they can live on, for example, by writing letters to loved ones. Team members can both share their own experiences and elicit stories from patients about special events in their lives to help young patients realize that they will live on in the memories of their family and friends.

## Advance Care Planning

Although the term *advance directive* is familiar to healthcare professionals, it may be meaningless to patients and their family members and friends. Patients with AIDS are less likely to discuss advance directives and life-limiting interventions with their physicians than other patient populations. Studies show that fewer than 50% of middle-aged patients receiving HIV care have documented advance care planning.[56] Advance care planning and goals of care should be addressed repeatedly during the course of illness, not only because many events along the way may alter patients' perspectives but also because patients may change their minds over time. Because the progression of late-stage AIDS is unpredictable, clinicians must be flexible and tolerant of the uncertainty and ambivalence that patients experience.[36]

When discussing future care management, clinicians should be aware of the patient's culture. For example, in the gay community, physician-assisted death has been a frequent topic of conversation, regardless of whether it becomes the patient's final choice. As the effectiveness of treatment has improved, however, assisted death and suicide are mentioned less frequently. African Americans are less likely to consider withdrawal or cessation of life-prolonging measures than other racial or ethnic groups.[36] Fears of being denied "best care" because of discrimination may result in a desire that everything be done.[57] In the Hispanic community, families may not want to include patients in discussions of future care management.[58]

Many people with HIV infection live in nontraditional unions. Although designating a healthcare proxy and completing an advance directive are important components of end-of-life care planning for all people, they are particularly important in nontraditional unions. A healthcare proxy can prevent conflicts between the family of origin and a nontraditional spouse or partner.

In addition to cultural factors in decision making, physicians also must also be aware that the persistent social stigma associated with AIDS and its concentration in vulnerable populations mean that patients and their families may view palliative care as somehow less than standard care.

See *UNIPAC 6* for more information on advance care planning.

### Rajesh's Case Concludes (continued from page 3)

You discuss Rajesh's illness and social circumstances with him and his husband. Rajesh has AIDS, as determined by the presence of HIV infection, CD4 cell count lower than 200 cells/mcL, and wasting. He has evidence of anal human papilloma virus (HPV) infection. Rajesh has not been forthright with his husband, who was previously unaware of Rajesh's HIV infection. Rajesh needs an opportunity to discuss his circumstances with his husband in an open, caring, and nonjudgmental manner. In addition, his husband's HIV status should be considered.

While you feel that hospice may be appropriate for Rajesh, and he may be eligible for this benefit (see **Table 3**), it is not yet time to admit Rajesh to the hospice program because he has not been evaluated by an HIV specialist and may respond positively to ART and prophylactic antibiotics. The usual treatment for wasting in HIV consists of proper nutrition, anabolic agents, treatment of opportunistic infections, and ART. The patient's blood dyscrasias could be related to opportunistic infections involving the bone marrow but are most likely secondary to the HIV infection itself. You call the internist and recommend that Rajesh be referred to an HIV specialist. You also share information about Rajesh's depression and his need to communicate with his husband and family.

Rajesh is referred to an HIV specialist, who prescribes ART and counsels Rajesh and his husband on HIV transmission and preexposure prophylaxis. His HIV viral load becomes undetectable, and his CD4 cell count increases by about 100 cells/mcL over the next 6 months. Rajesh's condition improves and he continues ART. After intensive counseling with his husband, Rajesh and his husband separate and he moves into his own apartment. His internist continues as his physician. Although asymptomatic, Rajesh's husband is discovered to be HIV positive and is referred for primary care for HIV.

No individual should be diagnosed as having end-stage AIDS unless an HIV specialist has conducted a thorough examination and reviewed the possible benefits of ART.

## Antiretroviral Therapy

Highly active ART suppresses HIV replication with the intent of producing both virologic and immunologic responses (see **Figure 1**). When therapy is effective, an individual's HIV viral load becomes undetectable (the virologic response), and the immune system can recover,

## Table 3. CMS HIV/AIDS Hospice Eligibility Guidelines[59]

Patients are considered to be in the terminal stage of their illness (life expectancy of 6 months or less) if they meet the following criteria (1 **and** 2 must be present; factors from 3 will add supporting documentation):

1. CD4+ count <25 cells/mcL or persistent (2 or more assays at least 1 month apart) viral load >100,000 copies/mL, plus **one** of the following:
   a. Central nervous system (CNS) lymphoma
   b. Untreated, or persistent despite treatment, wasting (loss of at least 33% lean body mass [Palmetto] or 10% lean body mass [CGS Administrators, LLC; National Government Services, Inc.])
   c. Mycobacterium avium complex bacteremia, untreated, unresponsive to treatment, or treatment refused
   d. Progressive multifocal leukoencephalopathy
   e. Systemic lymphoma, with advanced HIV infection and partial response to chemotherapy
   f. Visceral Kaposi's sarcoma unresponsive to therapy
   g. Renal failure in the absence of dialysis
   h. Cryptosporidium infection
   i. Toxoplasmosis, unresponsive to therapy.
2. Decreased performance status, as measured by the Karnofsky Performance Status (KPS) scale, of ≤50%
3. Documentation of the following factors will support eligibility for hospice care:
   a. Chronic persistent diarrhea for 1 year
   b. Persistent serum albumin <2.5 g/dL
   c. Concomitant, active substance abuse
   d. Age >50 years
   e. Absence of or resistance to effective antiretroviral, chemotherapeutic, and prophylactic drug therapy related specifically to HIV infection
   f. Advanced AIDS dementia complex
   g. Toxoplasmosis
   h. Congestive heart failure, symptomatic at rest
   i. Advanced liver disease (CGS Administrators, LLC; National Government Services, Inc.)

*LCD guidelines adapted from Indexes, Medicare Coverage Database, Centers for Medicare & Medicaid Services, https://www.cms.gov/medicare-coverage-database/indexes/lcd-contractor-index.aspx. Accessed May 31, 2017.*

*Note: Guidelines adapted here aggregate HIV-specific Local Coverage Determination (LCD) guidelines from the three Home Health and Hospice Medicare Administrative Contractors (MACs): CGS Administrators, LLC; National Government Services, Inc.; and Palmetto GBA. They do not include non-disease-specific guidelines that also appear in LCD guidelines. LCD guidelines for determining terminal status state that Medicare coverage for hospice care depends upon a physician's certification of an individual's prognosis of a life expectancy of 6 months or less, if the terminal illness runs its expected course and that some patients may not meet the guidelines provided in the LCDs yet still be appropriate for hospice care because of comorbities or rapid decline. Coverage for these patients may be approved if documentation of clinical factors supporting a 6-month-or-less life expectancy not included in the LCD guidelines is provided.*

# Figure 1. HIV Life Cycle and Drug Targets

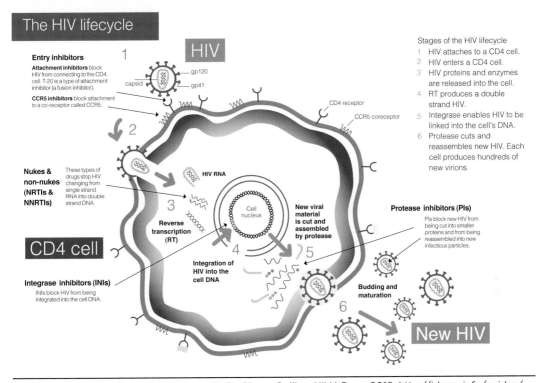

*Figure from Introduction to ART (Figure 5), by Simon Collins, HIV i-Base, 2016, http://i-base.info/guides/ starting/hiv-life-cycle. © 2017 by HIV i-Base (www.i-Base.info). Reproduced with permission.*

as assessed by an increase in CD4 lymphocytes (the immunologic response). When viral resistance occurs, an individual's HIV viral load will elevate despite the use of antiretroviral drugs, and he or she will experience progressive loss of both CD4 lymphocytes and immune competence.

Therapy may become ineffective for several reasons, including chronic nonadherence to medications, viral antimicrobial resistance, or the existence of other life-threatening conditions.[44,60-64] Patients with progressive loss of CD4 cells, total CD4 counts below 25 cells/mcL, and elevated HIV viral loads are at high risk of progressing to end-stage disease and death regardless of whether they are receiving ART.[65] In addition, those with fewer than 100 CD4 cells/mcL who are not receiving effective ART and appropriate opportunistic infection prophylaxis are at significant risk for developing AIDS-associated opportunistic infections that worsen prognosis.[66]

Individuals with low CD4 T-cell counts on treatment have increases in both AIDS-related and non-AIDS-related events, including cardiovascular, hepatic, renal, and cancer-related problems. ART does not appear to have reduced the incidence of some cancers, notably Hodgkin and non-Hodgkin lymphomas.[67,68] Although these lymphomas are frequently treatable,[69-71] people with HIV continue to die from them. Other cancers that have not lessened with ART are cervical cancer and anal cancer.

Potent combination ART is associated with numerous short- and long-term side effects. Effective management of the side effects is necessary to improve the patient's QOL. See **Table 4**[72,73] for a list of antiretroviral medications and side effects.

### Short-Term Side Effects of Antiretroviral Therapy

The most common short-term side effects of ART are similar to those associated with a wide variety of other medications. Nausea, anorexia, headache, and fatigue are common to all three classes of antiretrovirals: nucleoside reverse transcriptase inhibitors (NRTIs), nonnucleoside reverse transcriptase inhibitors (NNRTIs), and protease inhibitors (PIs). Nausea is a side effect of all ART agents. All three classes of antiretroviral medication can adversely affect liver function. Unfortunately some individuals with hepatitis C must discontinue ART because of an ART-associated acceleration of cirrhosis.

### Nucleoside Reverse Transcriptase Inhibitor Therapy

**Lactic Acidosis.** All NRTIs, like the antidiabetic agents phenformin and metformin, are associated with the potentially life-threatening syndrome lactic acidosis, characterized by fatigue, dyspnea, tachycardia, weight loss, nausea, vomiting, and abdominal pain.[74] In a 2011 study of 2,062 patients contributing 2,747 patient years (PY), the combined incidence of hyperlactatemia was 3.2/100 PY in those initiating stavudine-containing ART and 0.34/100 PY in those initiating zidovudine-containing ART. The analysis suggested that stavudine exposure, female sex, and higher body mass index are strong, independent predictors for developing hyperlactatemia. Patients with risk factors for lactic acidosis have less hyperlactatemia while on zidovudine- versus stavudine-containing ART. Switching patients from stavudine to zidovudine or alternative drugs improves outcomes.[75]

Other NRTIs such as didanosine also have been described as having this side effect.[73] The mechanism of lactic acidosis may involve mitochondrial toxicity due to the NRTI's poisoning polymerase gamma, the enzyme involved in replication of mitochondrial deoxyribonucleic acid (DNA).[76]

The NRTIs stavudine, didanosine, and zalcitabine (no longer available in the United States) are commonly associated with painful peripheral neuropathy. The neuropathy, like many other side effects of ART, often becomes more severe for individuals with advanced disease. Peripheral motor nerve dysfunction is a rare side effect also associated with these three NRTIs. Like other painful peripheral neuropathies, antiretroviral-related peripheral neuropathy can be treated with antidepressants, anticonvulsants, and opioid analgesics. Painful

## Table 4. Antiretroviral Medications and Side Effects

| Medication | Type of Agent | Side Effects |
|---|---|---|
| Abacavir | NRTI | Nausea, hypersensitivity reaction |
| Didanosine | NRTI | Pancreatitis, peripheral neuropathy, nausea, diarrhea, xerostomia |
| Emtricitabine | NRTI | Minimal side effects, nausea, rare CNS effects, lactic acidosis |
| Lamivudine | NRTI | Minimal side effects, nausea, rare CNS effects, lactic acidosis |
| Stavudine | NRTI | Peripheral neuropathy, lactic acidosis |
| Tenofovir | NRTI | Abdominal pain, diarrhea, nausea, vomiting, flatulence, rare neutropenia, elevated LFTs, hyperamylasemia |
| Zidovudine | NRTI | Anemia, neutropenia, headache, fatigue, anorexia, lactic acidosis, nausea |
| Delavirdine | NNRTI | Rash, nausea |
| Efavirenz | NNRTI | Nightmares, nausea, dizziness, rash, CNS changes |
| Etravirine | NNRTI | Rash, hypersensitivity reaction, nausea |
| Nevirapine | NNRTI | Rash, hepatitis, nausea, hypersensitivity reaction |
| Rilpivirine | NNRTI | Headaches, rash, depression, insomnia |
| Amprenavir | PI | Nausea, headache, diarrhea |
| Atazanavir | PI | Indirect hyperbilirubinemia, prolonged ECG PR interval |
| Darunavir | PI | Skin rash, Stevens-Johnson syndrome |
| Fosamprenavir | PI | Skin rash, diarrhea, nausea, headache |
| Indinavir | PI | Nephrolithiasis, abdominal pain, diarrhea, elevated LFTs, headache, dizziness, rash, altered taste, nausea, thrombocytopenia |
| Lopinavir/ritonavir | PI | Nausea, diarrhea, rash |
| Nelfinavir | PI | Diarrhea, nausea |
| Ritonavir (usually used as a "booster" for other PIs) | PI | Nausea, headache, diarrhea, circumoral paresthesia, elevated LFTs |

*Continued on page 14*

## Table 4. Antiretroviral Medications and Side Effects *(continued)*

| Medication | Type of Agent | Side Effects |
|---|---|---|
| Saquinavir | PI | Elevated LFTs, headache, nausea, diarrhea, CNS changes |
| Saquinavir [invirase] | PI | GI intolerance, elevated transaminases |
| Raltegravir Dolutegravir Elvitegravir | Integrase strand transfer inhibitors | Nausea, headache, diarrhea, CPK elevation |
| Enfuvirtide | Fusion inhibitor | Local reaction at injection site, bacterial pneumonia |
| Maraviroc | CCR5 antagonist | Abdominal pain, cough, dizziness, rash, hepatotoxicity, musculoskeletal symptoms |

*CCR5, C-C chemokine receptor type 5; CNS, central nervous system; CPK, creatine phosphokinase; ECG, electrocardiogram; LFT, liver function test; NNRTI, nonnucleoside reverse transcriptase inhibitor; NRTI, nucleoside reverse transcriptase inhibitor; PI, protease inhibitor. For updated information, see Johns Hopkins Guides at www.hopkinsguides.com/hopkins/ub/index/Johns_Hopkins_HIV_Guide/Drugs/Antiretrovirals.*

peripheral neuropathy in individuals who have HIV may result from many different causes, including medications and infections such as cytomegalovirus (CMV), herpes simplex, herpes zoster, and HIV itself.[77,78]

**Pancreatitis.** Didanosine, although infrequently used now, is associated with pancreatitis, which can be life threatening and can occur anytime during the course of didanosine therapy. Pancreatitis, which may occur before significant elevations of pancreatic amylase or lipase are detected, should be suspected if a patient complains of epigastric abdominal pain. All patients taking didanosine should be screened regularly for hyperamylasemia. Patients who develop clinical pancreatitis or significant elevations of serum amylase should discontinue their didanosine promptly. Although pancreatitis occurs much less frequently with other antiretroviral agents, it has been reported with all NRTIs and PIs except saquinavir, amprenavir, and lopinavir.

**Abacavir Hypersensitivity Reaction.** Abacavir, a very potent NRTI, is associated with a rare hypersensitivity reaction. This reaction, which has been reported in 3% to 5% of individuals taking the drug, is characterized by multiple symptoms in several organ systems. Individuals usually experience three or more of the following symptoms: nausea, abdominal pain, fever, rash, headache, cough, fatigue, and malaise. The symptoms typically increase with each subsequent dose of abacavir. The hypersensitivity reaction most often occurs in the first 6 weeks of therapy. A screening test, the HLA 5701, helps predict patients who have high risk for the reaction. Because an abacavir hypersensitivity reaction may mimic other syndromes (eg, infection, immune reconstitution inflammatory syndrome, and other drug reactions), patients who think they are experiencing a hypersensitivity reaction should contact their healthcare professionals immediately. If abacavir therapy is discontinued because of an actual or suspected hypersensitivity reaction, it can never be resumed. *Reinstituting abacavir therapy for patients who have experienced a hypersensitivity reaction can be life-threatening.* For this reason, an expert clinician must promptly evaluate any patient suspected of abacavir hypersensitivity. If an HIV specialist confirms that a patient has the signs and symptoms of abacavir hypersensitivity reaction, it should be discontinued immediately.

### Nonnucleoside Reverse Transcriptase Inhibitor Therapy

**Maculopapular Rash.** NNRTI therapy is associated with an itchy red maculopapular rash in 5% to 20% of individuals. Unlike many other drug-related eruptions, an NNRTI-associated rash may involve the face and hands. The rash usually is time limited and can be treated with corticosteroids and antihistamines. Pretreatment with corticosteroids has not been shown to prevent the rash.[79]

**Hepatitis.** NNRTI therapy also is associated with hepatitis, which rarely is life threatening.[80] Some evidence indicates that people coinfected with hepatitis C are at greater risk for developing frank hepatitis when taking NNRTIs and PIs rather than NRTIs.

**Mood and Cognitive Disorders and Sleep Disturbances.** The NNRTI efavirenz is associated with mood and cognitive disorders and sleep disturbances during the first 2 to 3 weeks of therapy. Patients describe vivid dreams and nightmares in the early stages of treatment. Many also experience dizziness, so patients are usually directed to take the medication at bedtime. Education and reassurance prior to and during early therapy are usually all that is needed to help patients cope with these transient side effects until they resolve.

The NNRTIs efavirenz and nevirapine also induce the cytochrome P450 3A4 system. Thus, they can lower levels of many coadministered medications, including PIs and methadone.

### Protease Inhibitor Therapy

The most common short-term side effects of PIs are diarrhea and nausea, which usually can be managed with typical antidiarrheals and antiemetics. The addition of calcium to nelfinavir can alleviate diarrhea in some patients. Indinavir is associated with renal calculi, which can be prevented by drinking 1.5 L of water daily. Individuals taking indinavir also may experience flank pain similar to renal colic but without documented renal calculi. Atazanavir is associated with asymptomatic elevation of bilirubin.

### Fusion Inhibitors: Enfuvirtide

Enfuvirtide is an injectable fusion inhibitor administered in a dose of 90 mg subcutaneously twice a day. Side effects include local injection site reactions, increased pneumonias, and hypersensitivity reactions.

## Integrase Strand Transfer Inhibitors

Raltegravir, an integrase strand transfer inhibitor, was approved in 2007. It is used in a dose of 400 mg twice daily. Potential side effects include nausea, headache, fever, and rhabdomyolysis with increased creatine phosphokinase (CPK).

## CCR5 Antagonists

The medication maraviroc was approved in 2007 and is known to be effective only for patients who have the R5 virus. It is a substrate of CYP3A; therefore, its level is increased by PI drugs such as ritonavir. It is used in a dose of 150 mg twice daily. Side effects include abdominal pain, cough, upper respiratory infection, and hepatotoxicity.

## *Long-Term Complications of Antiretroviral Therapy*
### Lipodystrophy Syndrome

The most commonly recognized long-term complications associated with ART are insulin resistance, abnormalities of serum lipids, and derangements of fat distribution, collectively described as *lipodystrophy syndrome*. When first recognized in 1996, lipodystrophy syndrome was attributed to PI therapy, and patients with lipodystrophy were described as having a *protease paunch*.[81] Rigorous investigation indicates, however, that most of the manifestations of lipodystrophy syndrome are associated with all antiretroviral medications.[82-85] In fact, lipodystrophy and lipoatrophy have been described for patients with HIV who have never taken ART. Nevertheless, PIs can accelerate NRTI-associated lipodystrophy and lipoatrophy.[86] Discontinuing ART appears to arrest its development, but no therapy has been shown to reliably reverse lipodystrophy.

The fat distribution abnormalities include lipoatrophy (ie, wasting of fat in the limbs, face, and buttocks) and lipodystrophy (ie, fat accumulation in the dorsal spine [buffalo hump], trunk [fat accumulation is predominantly visceral adipose tissue], and breasts).

### Metabolic Complications

Metabolic complications of ART and long-term HIV infection, such as hyperlipidemia and glucose intolerance, place individuals who have HIV at increased risk for atherosclerotic disease.[87] The risk of atherosclerosis increases for individuals who smoke, have hypertension, and have a positive family history of atherosclerosis.

Hyperlipidemia is associated with most PI- and efavirenz-based ART regimens. The drugs atazanavir, nevirapine, etravirine, and maraviroc are less commonly associated with hyperlipidemia. Since 1996 insulin resistance has been reported with ART.[88] PIs have been shown to block glucose transport into cells, raising blood glucose levels.[89] Evidence indicates that PIs can induce insulin resistance for individuals who are not infected with HIV.[90]

The accumulation of visceral adipose tissue may be associated with insulin resistance and hyperlipidemia. The triad of truncal obesity, insulin resistance, and hyperlipidemia is similar to syndrome X, an inherited disorder of lipid metabolism that increases the risk of developing atherosclerotic cardiovascular disease. Anecdotal reports of sudden deaths attributable to atherosclerotic cardiovascular disease are increasing in programs that treat patients with HIV.

In addition, there are reports of QT prolongation and Stevens-Johnson syndrome caused by several antiretroviral agents.[73]

## Clinical Situation

### Juan

Juan has long-standing HIV infection. He was exposed to HIV during heterosexual encounters with sex workers in Asia. Juan has been on ART with tenofovir, emtricitabine, and raltegravir as initial therapy for 4 years. He has an undetectable viral load and a CD4 cell count of 655 cells/mcL. Recently Juan developed lung cancer, which was unresponsive to surgery, chemotherapy, and radiation therapy, and he is referred to your hospice program with progressive lung cancer. He is weak and somewhat short of breath. Juan complains of tingling pain in his hands and feet that has been present since the last round of chemotherapy. You take his medical history and perform a medical examination. The tingling in Juan's hands and feet began after chemotherapy for cancer and is now present all the time. The chemotherapy has also left him anorexic. He has no other complaints except for mild dyspnea on exertion.

On examination, Juan weighs 165 lb (normal adult weight for him is 172 lb). He has some supraclavicular adenopathy on both sides and diminished breath sounds at the right-lung base. His liver is enlarged. He has diminished sensation to light touch and pinprick in all his distal extremities.

 What is the most appropriate management at this time?

*Case continues on page 33*

## Managing Common Symptoms of HIV/AIDS

Cicely Saunders, OM DBE FRCS FRCP FRCN, founder of modern-day hospice care at St. Christopher's in London, introduced the concept of *total pain*,[91] which provides a model for symptom management. She recognized that each complaint includes physical, emotional, and spiritual components. In keeping with this principle, vigilant listening and history taking must be an integral part of medical and nursing care and social service because specific symptoms and questions may have deeper meanings for patients and their family members than other symptoms.[92] For example, a patient may believe that a symptom is God's punishment. The patient may be addressing other HIV-related issues, such as guilt associated with engaging in high-risk behaviors or transmitting the disease to children. These and similar concerns can exacerbate any symptom. When a symptom seems particularly difficult to control, it may be useful to ask the patient questions such as "What does the pain (or nausea or shortness of breath) mean to you?" and "What do you think is causing this symptom?"

A number of studies have demonstrated remarkable consistency in the prevalence of common symptoms primarily in, but not limited to, patients with advanced HIV infection.[34,93-98] The results of these studies are summarized in **Table 5**. These symptoms include a mixture of physical and mental health symptoms (eg, pain, anorexia, fatigue, anxiety, depression, nausea and vomiting, diarrhea). Later studies have shown that patients with HIV still have serious symptom burdens at the time of diagnosis (pain, 11%-76%; weight loss, 8%-89%; fever, 32%-89%; diarrhea, 6%-54%; anxiety, 36%-95%; and depression, 18%-47%).[99] The best symptom management intervention may be disease specific (eg, ART, therapy for opportunistic infections, antineoplastic therapy) and sometimes nonspecific and supportive. Consistent with the basic principles of palliative care, the decision whether and how to treat specific symptoms should be made within the context of the intended goals of care. For example, one may forgo the exhaustive search for the cause of a fever in a patient with terminal disease in favor of treating symptoms and providing comfort measures.

## Fatigue

Fatigue, or asthenia, is an often overlooked and poorly described symptom of HIV infection, yet it may be the most prevalent of all symptoms affecting QOL.[97] Studies using a variety of methodologies have documented a high prevalence of fatigue, with rates ranging from 48% to 95%.[100] Although fatigue generally is considered a reactive state of tiredness or weariness, clinically significant fatigue refers to an inability to sustain activities of daily living (ADLs) regardless of required level of activity.

Fatigue can occur throughout the illness trajectory and usually worsens as death approaches. Like other symptoms, fatigue can have physical, psychological, and spiritual causes. Anemia, malnutrition, AIDS dementia, hypogonadism, HIV myopathy, unrelieved pain, HIV medications, chemotherapies, immunotherapies, radiation therapy, opportunistic infections, and malignancies all can contribute to fatigue.[101] Later studies have shown that depression, anxiety, unemployment, stressful life events, and poor social support are important contributors, as well.[102-105] Because so many factors may cause or contribute to fatigue, physicians may find it difficult to offer a clear explanation for the symptom.

Physical examination and laboratory studies can help distinguish the multiple etiologies of fatigue. See **Table 6** for treatable causes of fatigue in HIV infection. As with any symptom, successful management begins with a careful evaluation guided by potential etiology.

Successful management involves treatments tailored to the patient's prognosis and full participation by members of an interdisciplinary team (IDT).[103] Fatigue management strategies typically are divided into those aimed at treating the underlying cause of fatigue and those aimed at treating fatigue directly. While fatigue is being evaluated, a physical therapy

## Table 5. Prevalence of Symptoms Experienced by Patients with AIDS[34,93-98,100]

| Symptom | Percentage Range |
|---|---|
| Fatigue or lack of energy | 48-95 |
| Weight loss | 37-91 |
| Pain | 29-76 |
| Anorexia | 26-51 |
| Insomnia | 21-50 |
| Cough | 19-60 |
| Nausea or vomiting | 17-43 |
| Dyspnea or respiratory symptoms | 15-48 |
| Depression or sadness | 15-40 |
| Diarrhea | 11-32 |
| Constipation | 10-29 |

*Note: Data are based on available descriptive studies of patients with AIDS, predominantly in patients with late-stage disease, 1990-2002.*

## Table 6. Treatable Causes of Fatigue in HIV Disease

| | |
|---|---|
| **F** | Fear of the unknown |
| **A** | Anemia, adrenal or testosterone insufficiency |
| **T** | Treatments given (lactic acidosis), thyroid inactive, tumor |
| **I** | Insomnia, inactivity, infection (occult *mycobacterium avium* complex, abscess) |
| **G** | General metabolic |
| **U** | Uncontrolled disease: HIV, other organs, undernourished |
| **E** | Emotions (anxiety or depression) |

consultation and exercise recommendations can promote a sense of independence and control for ambulatory patients and family members. Asking the patient to keep a diary of energy levels throughout the day and sleep patterns during the day and night may reveal important information. Frequent, brief visits with members of the healthcare team can provide emotional support and reassurance. Activities such as reading, listening to music, and enjoying a hobby can help patients retain a sense of creativity and usefulness. Rearranging the patient's room to remove impediments to activity can be helpful.

In addition to ART, pharmacologic management is directed at the cause of the symptom. Depending on the patient's prognosis and hemoglobin level, a blood transfusion may be appropriate and may partially relieve fatigue. Fatigue associated with simple dehydration may be corrected with increased oral intake or a short course of hypodermoclysis or intravenous fluids. Testosterone injections or gel may be helpful for men with HIV and low testosterone levels. Psychostimulants such as methylphenidate, armodafinil, or modafinil can result in improved functioning and increased energy.[106,107] Most patients tolerate these medications well without significant risk of misuse, even for substance users. Sympathomimetic side effects can generally be avoided by using low dosages and titrating upward gradually.[3] The use of progesterone therapies has not been well supported for noncancer cachexia, although they may have a role in appetite stimulation.[108]

## Gastrointestinal Symptoms

Nausea, dysphagia, odynophagia, and diarrhea are common gastrointestinal symptoms experienced by patients with end-stage AIDS. Nausea is one of the most common symptoms associated with HIV infection and is a side effect of all classes of antiretroviral agents. For a full discussion of the etiology and management of nausea, see *UNIPAC 4*.

### Odynophagia and Dysphagia

A history of dysphagia (difficulty swallowing) or odynophagia (painful swallowing) for a patient with HIV/AIDS should raise concerns regarding esophagitis. Patients who have not attained immune reconstitution with ART or who have a CD4 count of less than 100 cells/mcL are at particularly high risk.[109] The most common causes of esophagitis in this population include *Candida*, herpes simplex virus, CMV, and idiopathic (aphthous) esophageal ulcers.

Given the high probability of *Candida* as the etiology of esophagitis before ART,[110,111] many physicians will empirically treat patients with a course of fluconazole.[112] If symptoms persist, endoscopy and biopsy are necessary.[113] Although the presence of oropharyngeal candidiasis can predict the presence of esophageal candidiasis, the converse is not true. In one study, the presence of esophageal candidiasis without oropharyngeal candidiasis approached 20%.[114] When odynophagia is the most prominent symptom, especially without the presence of oropharyngeal candidiasis, one should suspect ulcerative esophagitis. The ulcers can be idiopathic (aphthous) ulcers or secondary to herpes simplex or CMV infection. Chronic esophageal candidiasis also can lead to ulcerations, which harbor CMV. For patients receiving ART, gastroesophageal reflux disease (GERD), gastric ulcers, and *Helicobacter pylori* infections are more commonly being found.[115] Idiopathic esophageal ulcers often respond to short courses of prednisone. If presumptive prednisone treatment is ineffective, a course of famciclovir or a similar antiherpes medicine may be helpful. Thalidomide also is an option for refractory ulcers. For patients with end-stage AIDS, a mixture of topical viscous lidocaine and an antacid may be helpful.[116] See **Table 7** for medications to treat oropharyngeal and esophageal diseases in this population.

## Table 7. Medications for Treating Oropharyngeal and Esophageal Disease

| Condition | Symptom | Medication | Comments |
|---|---|---|---|
| Oral or esophageal candidiasis | Altered taste, dysphagia | Fluconazole or itraconazole | May require dosages up to 800 mg/day if resistance develops |
| Azole-resistant oral or esophageal candidiasis | Altered taste, dysphagia | Amphotericin B suspension, amphotericin B IV, or caspofungin anidulafungin micafungin | IV administration; requires premedication with acetaminophen, 650 mg PO; diphenhydramine, 50 mg IV; and hydrocortisone, 50 mg IV<br><br>Meperidine, 25 mg slow IV push for shaking chills |
| Aphthous ulcers | Pain in mouth, odynophagia | Prednisone or thalidomide | Thalidomide can cause rash, sedation, or peripheral neuropathy |
| Herpetic ulcers | Pain in mouth, odynophagia | Famciclovir, valacyclovir, or acyclovir | |
| CMV ulcers | Odynophagia | Ganciclovir, valganciclovir, or foscarnet | Use in biopsy-diagnosed cases; watch for serious drug interactions |

*CMV, cytomegalovirus; IV, intravenous; PO, by mouth*

**Diarrhea**

For patients with HIV, diarrhea can be a significant source of morbidity. Infectious pathogens, malignancies, and medications all should be considered as possible etiologies.[117]

With regard to infectious etiologies, the incidence of infectious diarrhea has declined with the advent of ART.[118,119] The pathogens associated with diarrheal disease vary with the degree of immunosuppression. Pathogens, which cause disease in normal hosts, certainly can cause diarrhea in those infected with HIV. In patients with more severe immunosuppression, less virulent organisms can cause disease. For example, *Cryptosporidium parvum* can cause significant diarrhea in those with a CD4 count less than 180 cells/mcL. More importantly, the parasite can be quite difficult, if not impossible, to eradicate. In those with more severe immunosuppression, *Mycobacterium avium* complex can cause bowel infiltration, fever, and malabsorption.

With noninfectious etiologies, medications are a common cause of diarrhea. These can include medications to prevent opportunistic infections or even ART itself. In those with greater constitutional symptoms, malignancies such as lymphoma or Kaposi's sarcoma should be considered.[120]

For those who present with diarrhea, a complete history should be taken and a physical exam conducted. Particular attention should be given to recent medication changes, HIV disease status, and constitutional symptoms. Depending on the severity of symptoms and goals of care, initial evaluation should include stool examination for bacterial culture, *Clostridium difficile* toxin assay, and examination for ova and parasites. An acid-fast smear also should be requested to look for *Cryptosporidium, Isospora,* and *Cyclospora.* Finally, if disseminated *Mycobacterium avium* complex (MAC) infection is a diagnostic consideration, blood cultures should also be obtained. If these studies do not lead to a diagnosis, endoscopy and biopsy, which are diagnostic in 30% to 70% of pathogen-negative cases,[121] can be considered.

Management might include presumptive treatment with a broad-spectrum antibiotic (eg, metronidazole, 250 mg to 500 mg three times daily), and antidiarrheal medications may be all that is necessary. The US Food and Drug Administration has approved crofelemer (125 mg by mouth twice daily) to relieve symptoms of diarrhea in patients with HIV/AIDS who are receiving antiretroviral therapy. Additional treatment should be guided by the results of the workup and goals of care.[122]

Abdominal pain in end-stage AIDS occurs for various reasons. Medication side effects, infectious gastroenteritis, CMV enteritis, HIV enteropathy, visceral neoplasms, and disseminated MAC can cause cramping, bloating, diarrhea, and pain. Individuals with stable or advanced HIV disease may benefit from disease-specific treatment for these conditions. However, those with end-stage disease should be treated with typical palliative medications, including opioid analgesics, antispasmodics, and antidiarrheal agents. Ketorolac or corticosteroids may be helpful for short-term treatment of the pain of intraabdominal MAC. Patients with advanced disease may require a strict bowel regimen designed to promote regular bowel movements and minimize the symptoms of enteropathy.

### Neuropsychiatric Disorders

Neuropsychiatric disorders are common for individuals with HIV infection. HIV is neurotropic, infecting the central nervous system (CNS) early in the course of disease. The neurotropic effects of HIV and the side effects of some medications may cause or exacerbate mood disorders, dementia, organic and delusional disorders, and delirium. In addition, preexisting psychiatric conditions, substance abuse, and social isolation can further exacerbate these problems. These disorders may occur at any stage of disease[123] and significantly affect care near the end of life. Although recent findings demonstrate that patients with psychiatric disorders have a greater likelihood of being prescribed ART,[124] studies have clearly shown that patients with neuropsychiatric conditions have poorer outcomes and receive less benefit from ART. Psychiatric symptoms are among the most difficult to manage, and the full extent of their impact on a patient's QOL cannot be underestimated. Several studies have identified statistics that give cause for concern.

Mood disorders, particularly depression and anxiety, were present in more than 48% of a cohort of 2,864 patients with HIV using data from the HIV Cost and Services Utilization

Study.[125] Depression correlates with low self-esteem,[126] increased disease factors, and fewer personal and social supports. African American women are at higher risk for depression than other populations.[127] One study by the CDC showed that women from socially and economically disadvantaged environments—both those who were infected with HIV and those who were not infected with HIV—experienced higher levels of depression.[30]

Because of the scarcity of community-based residential treatment programs, patients with severe psychiatric disorders may be admitted to long-term care facilities earlier and live there longer than those with other HIV-related diagnoses.[128] In addition to the difficulty of coping with HIV/AIDS alone, neuropsychiatric conditions place a profound strain on the individual, his or her caregivers, and the family. Consequently treatment adherence can suffer.

## HIV-Associated Neurological Syndromes

HIV-associated neurological syndromes can be classified as primary HIV neurological disease, secondary or opportunistic neurological disease, and treatment-related neurological disease (such as immune reconstitution inflammatory syndrome).[129] The mortality associated with CNS complications and opportunistic infections is still high in patients who are untreated or unaware of their HIV infection.[130]

**Primary HIV Neurological Disease.** HIV-associated neurocognitive disorder (HAND) is the most common CNS manifestation of HIV. It is a chronic neurodegenerative condition characterized by cognitive, central motor, and behavioral abnormalities. Although HAND can affect any neuropsychological domain, the most commonly reported deficits are in attention and concentration, psychomotor speed, memory and learning, information processing, and executive functioning. Language and visuospatial abilities are relatively unaffected.[131] Aggressive forms of HAND were prevalent before the advent of ART and were viewed as a precursor to death. Before the introduction of combination ART, two-thirds of patients infected with HIV were expected to demonstrate eventual signs of HIV dementia.[128] This can still be seen in developing countries, in individuals in late stages of the disease, and in those who have refused ART or for whom ART has failed as a treatment.

Such presentations are uncommon for patients successfully treated with ART. These individuals can, however, present with a milder, less lethal form of HAND that progresses more slowly.[132,133] Caring for such patients can be difficult; although they may appear cognitively intact during an office visit and may perform well on the Mini-Mental State Examination, they may have difficulty processing and retaining the content of discussions with the physician. Such patients are likely to pose clinical and ethical management concerns requiring careful analysis from the viewpoint of the patient, the staff, and other caregivers.[34]

**Secondary or Opportunistic Neurological Disease.** Secondary or opportunistic neurological diseases can present in patients with HIV. These can include CNS lymphoma and opportunistic infections such as progressive multifocal leukoencephalopathy (PML), CMV, cryptococcal meningitis, and cerebral toxoplasmosis. Although the incidence of these infections is decreasing, the mortality after such a diagnosis remains high.[134]

PML is a demyelinating disease of the CNS caused by the John Cunningham virus (JC virus). Most cases occur in the presence of severe immunosuppression (CD4 count less than 100 cells/mcL). Patients often present with a subacute onset of mental status change and focal neurological symptoms.[135,136] No specific treatment for PML exists; however, ART has improved the course of the disease and decreased mortality.

A member of the herpes virus family, CMV infection typically presents in individuals with CD4 counts less than 50 cells/mcL. The virus can infect the CNS and peripheral nervous system as well as visceral organs.[137] Presenting signs and symptoms depend on the areas affected. CMV retinitis affects the vision of patients with advanced HIV/AIDS. It also is associated with immune reconstitution after ART is started. Treatment often is initiated with agents such as ganciclovir or foscarnet but can be discontinued after patients have immune recovery and quiescent retinitis.[138]

An encapsulated yeast, *Cryptococcus neoformans* often presents as an infection in patients with a CD4 count less than 100 cells/mcL. The most common presentation is a subacute meningoencephalitis with malaise, headache, and fever.[139] Immediate treatment is essential to prevent additional neurological injury and mortality. Initial treatment includes amphotericin B and flucytosine, possibly followed by fluconazole. Patients with increased intracranial pressure may require repeated lumbar punctures for palliation.[140]

*Toxoplasma gondii* is an intracellular protozoan pathogen. Associated with CD4 counts less than 200 cells/mcL,[141] infection with toxoplasmosis often presents with fever, headache, cognitive dysfunction, and seizures.[142] The typical neuroimages reveal multiple contrast-enhancing ring lesions with surrounding edema. The initial treatment includes pyrimethamine, sulfadiazine, and leucovorin.

Finally, primary CNS lymphoma often presents with CD4 counts less than 100 cells/mcL. Associated with prior Epstein Barr virus infection, the majority of these lymphomas are high-grade diffuse B-cell lymphomas. Treatments include radiation therapy, ART, and chemotherapy. Outcomes are better for patients with a better performance status,[143] but treatment can result in residual neurological impairment.

**Treatment-Related Neurological Disease.** The immune reconstitution inflammatory syndrome (IRIS) refers to a group of syndromes characterized by clinical worsening usually occurring within the first 4 to 8 weeks after the patient begins ART.[144] The reconstituted immune system generates an inflammatory response resulting in either a worsening of a known underlying infection or the unmasking of a subclinical indolent infection (eg, CMV, PML, toxoplasmosis). Risk factors for this syndrome include taking ART for the first time, a CD4 count of less than 50 cells/mcL, and active or subclinical opportunistic infections.[145,146] The risks of developing IRIS can be decreased by starting ART early in the course of the illness or by reducing antigenic burden with antimicrobial treatment for opportunistic infections before starting ART.[147]

## Evaluation and Management

Early in the course of illness, patients with HIV who show signs of organic mood disturbances or personality changes should be investigated with a computed tomography (CT) scan of the head or magnetic resonance imaging (MRI) and lumbar puncture to rule out treatable causes. It is important to remember that ART alone can result in neurocognitive disturbances. Antiretroviral agents such as efavirenz, saquinavir, and lamivudine can precipitate bad dreams, acute psychiatric episodes, and even severe suicidal ideation. Medication side effects should be suspected when a patient presents with changes in personality or mood disorders after recently beginning a new medication. Methadone-dependent patients may experience acute withdrawal symptoms with the initiation of the NNRTIs efavirenz and nevirapine and the PI ritonavir, all of which increase the metabolism of methadone.

In all cases, treatment of the underlying etiology may improve cognitive function. As patients become more debilitated, further evaluation may become too stressful, at which time symptoms should be treated empirically.

### Pain Management for Patients with HIV

Pain is common in patients with HIV,[148] and its management should follow the same basic principles followed for other patient populations (see *UNIPAC 3*). However, pain experienced by patients with HIV/AIDS does present unique challenges:

- With a focus on ART and disease-specific therapy, pain experienced by patients with AIDS tends to be underdiagnosed and undertreated.
- Because of the complex needs of patients who may have a history of substance abuse, healthcare providers may be reluctant to prescribe opioid analgesics to these patients.[149]
- Neuropathic pain syndromes are quite common in patients with AIDS. Given the longer survival of patients treated with ART, the prevalence of these syndromes has increased.
- Many medications used to treat HIV/AIDS can potentially have adverse interactions with the medications used for pain management. For example, methadone is metabolized by the hepatic microsomal enzyme CYP 3A4. The PI class of HIV antiretroviral agents increases the amount and activity of this enzyme system. As a result, methadone levels can decrease enough to result in inadequate analgesia or opioid withdrawal.
- Pain is the most common reason for referral to HIV palliative medicine clinics[98] and is associated with substantially increased odds of impairment in physical function.[108]

Given the need to balance curative therapy with effective symptom management, pain management for patients with HIV/AIDS remains as challenging as it was before the arrival of ART.[3,150,151]

### Rashes in HIV Disease

Dermatologic manifestations in HIV/AIDS patients act as markers of disease progression.[152,153] Two itchy red rashes are common in patients with AIDS: seborrheic dermatitis and eosinophilic folliculitis. Seborrheic dermatitis typically involves the skin folds of the face and the intertriginous region. It is red, itchy, and flaky and is associated with dandruff. Effective treatments include keratolytics, antifungals, topical corticosteroids, or a brief course of systemic corticosteroids.

Eosinophilic folliculitis involves a rash with discrete erythematous papules on the limbs and trunk. For want of a better term, the pruritic papular eruption[154] is often referred to as *itchy red-bump disease.* Usually patients have tried antihistamines and topical steroids without relief. Biopsy may not be helpful because it frequently documents a perivascular infiltrate of eosinophils and lymphocytes. The differential diagnosis includes acne, bacterial folliculitis, atopic dermatitis, pityrosporum folliculitis, papular urticaria, scabies, and drug eruption.[155] In addition to antihistamines and topical steroids, successful treatment has been reported with itraconazole, retinoids, doxycycline,[156] metronidazole, and phototherapy.[157]

Some dermatologic disorders may be ameliorated with reconstitution of the immune system using ART. On the other hand, some skin diseases flare temporarily when ART is initiated.[158] Unless a true drug allergy is suspected, ART does not need to be stopped.

## HIV Wasting Syndrome and Anorexia

*Wasting,* defined as weight loss of 10% or greater from baseline, and unintentional weight loss are harbingers of a poor outcome for individuals infected with HIV. Weight loss and wasting are independent predictors of mortality in patients with HIV infection.[159] Studies indicate that people die when they reach 66% of ideal body weight.[160]

The causes of wasting and anorexia in patients with HIV infection are multifactorial. They include hypogonadism, malnutrition, malabsorption, and infection. Many of these causes can be specifically addressed for individuals on successful ART.

Initiation of ART with subsequent viral suppression among therapy-naïve patients increases weight and lean body mass over a relatively short duration of 16 weeks.[161] Nutritional support and education also can have a positive impact.

Successful pharmacologic interventions can include corticosteroids, dronabinol, megestrol acetate, oxandrolone, testosterone, other anabolic steroids, recombinant growth hormone, and thalidomide.[162] These therapies have been associated with increased weight, appetite, energy, sense of well-being, lean muscle mass, and even survival. Before these medications are instituted, the following observations should be considered[163]:

- Anabolic agents and growth hormone have been associated with greater increases in lean muscle mass than the other classes of agents.[164] Some medications (eg, oxandrolone, anabolic steroids), however, may be associated with hepatotoxicity. Growth hormone is associated with the possibility of insulin resistance, swelling, and joint pain.
- Megestrol is a potent appetite stimulant and can be effective for individuals with a variety of end-stage illnesses, including AIDS. The weight gained with megestrol is primarily fat, however,[165] which limits its usefulness for individuals on successful ART. Because megestrol can cause glucose intolerance and adrenal suppression, its administration should be

tapered when treatment is discontinued. Megestrol also is associated with an increased risk of venous thromboembolism.

- Dronabinol, an active ingredient in marijuana, is an effective appetite stimulant, but its psychotropic effects can limit its usefulness. This can be of particular concern for patients suffering from neuropsychiatric disorders. Individuals with past positive experiences with marijuana often tolerate dronabinol better than other patients.

- Oral corticosteroids, such as prednisone, also are effective appetite stimulants for people with end-stage AIDS.

For more information about anorexia, see *UNIPAC 4.*

## Issues of Special Interest for HIV Patients at the End of Life

### *Malignancy*

HIV/AIDS is associated with an increased chance of malignancy. Before ART, malignancies accounted for fewer than 10% of all deaths among HIV patients.[166,167] With the advent of ART and longer survival for patients, malignancies are responsible for a greater proportion of deaths of patients with HIV/AIDS.

The cancer burden and types of cancers changed dramatically in the United States from 1991 to 2005. An increase in non-AIDS-defining cancers is attributed to increased survival because of ART and the increased cancer risk in an aging population. In particular, the incidence of lung cancer, anal cancer, liver cancer, and Hodgkin disease has increased. These increased risks are estimated to be 3-fold for lung cancer, 29-fold for anal cancer, 5-fold for liver cancer, and 11-fold for Hodgkin disease.[168] Reproductive cancers in women, including cancers of the cervix and vulva, also have increased. Because of the rise in these malignancies and the unique challenges of HIV, there is a continuing need to enroll individuals with HIV in clinical trials.[168]

### Kaposi's Sarcoma

Principally a disease affecting men, Kaposi's sarcoma is a low-grade soft-tissue sarcoma of vascular origin associated with human herpes virus 8 (HHV-8). Early in the HIV epidemic, Kaposi's sarcoma was noted in 20% to 30% of homosexual men with HIV infection. This disease has a variable course, ranging from an asymptomatic clinical finding to explosive growth resulting in significant morbidity and mortality. Skin involvement is characteristic, but extracutaneous spread is common. Incidence has decreased substantially since the mid 1990s.[168]

Kaposi's sarcoma can be devastating for people with HIV because the lesions are outwardly visible markers of disease. The obvious signs may cause other people to avoid physical contact because they fear contagion; however, the disease is not spread in this manner. Use of ART has been reported to cause remission of early Kaposi's sarcoma in up to 60% of patients,[169] but it may require aggressive palliation in end-stage disease. When an extremity is involved, lymphatic drainage is eventually impaired, and lymphedema (more indurated than in breast cancer) may become quite painful. Initially radiation and chemotherapy can be quite helpful.[170]

Diuretics and elevation may give symptomatic relief in the early stages. Steroids have been used to reduce swelling, but their effectiveness is poorly documented. In most cases, opioids are required for pain control.

## Non-Hodgkin Lymphoma

For AIDS patients, the incidence of non-Hodgkin lymphoma increases with progressively worsening immunosuppression. Unlike the incidence of cancers of the lung, liver, anus, and cervix, the incidence of non-Hodgkin lymphoma, along with Kaposi's sarcoma, has decreased significantly in the ART era.[171] Approximately 70% to 90% of these lymphomas are intermediate or high grade (diffuse large B-cell or Burkitt's-like lymphomas).[172] Approximately two-thirds of HIV-positive patients with systemic non-Hodgkin lymphoma present with extranodal disease, with the gastrointestinal tract being the most commonly involved. Overall, however, the incidence of non-Hodgkin lymphoma has decreased in population of patients with HIV. Although prognosis for non-Hodgkin lymphoma has improved since ART was introduced, it is still poor despite high initial response rates to chemotherapy.[173] The median survival is less than 1 year, with the majority of patients dying from disease progression or other AIDS-related complications.

## Hodgkin Lymphoma

A number of epidemiologic studies have demonstrated that the risk of Hodgkin lymphoma is 3 to 18 times higher for patients with AIDS.[168,174-179] CD4 count, hepatitis B, age, and ART therapy all seem to be independent predictors for the incidence of this and other malignancies.[180]

The pathological spectrum of Hodgkin lymphoma in the United States differs between patients infected with HIV and those who do not have HIV. The majority of patients infected with HIV have the mixed cellularity subtype rather than nodular sclerosis, which is the most common type in other populations.[181]

Compared with patients without HIV infection, patients with HIV usually present with systemic B symptoms (eg, fever, weight loss, nocturnal sweats). In addition, widely disseminated extranodal disease is seen in 75% to 90% of patients at presentation.[182]

Before ART, combination chemotherapy was able to induce complete remission in a variable percentage of HIV-positive patients with Hodgkin lymphoma. The median survival, however, ranged between 12 and 18 months. Because of chemotherapy-induced neutropenia, death often was due to bacterial or opportunistic infection.[183-185]

Since the introduction of ART, the incidence of Hodgkin lymphoma in patients with HIV does not appear to have decreased.[186] There is some evidence, however, that patients present with less advanced disease. In addition, the combination of ART with intensive chemotherapy suggests improved survival.[187-189]

## Anogenital Malignancy

The incidence of both anal squamous intraepithelial lesions and anal cancer in men and women with HIV has increased significantly. The risk has increased 29-fold for anal cancer in this population.[168] Risk factors for the development of anogenital malignancies include concurrent human papilloma virus (HPV) infection, receptive anal intercourse, and increased number of lifetime sexual partners.[190-192] Unfortunately the widespread use of ART does not appear to have reduced the incidence of either anal squamous intraepithelial lesions or anal cancer in men who are HIV positive who have sex with men.[193] Educating patients and eliminating risk factors remain critical to prevention. Guidelines for the use of anal cytologic screening are being developed.[194]

## CNS Lymphoma

Associated with a greater degree of immunosuppression than non-Hodgkin lymphoma, the majority of CNS lymphomas are large cell or large-cell immunoblastic types of B-cell origin. The treatment for primary CNS lymphoma involves radiation combined with steroids. Prognosis remains poor, but it is better in patients receiving ART and in those with a Karnofsky performance status (KPS) score greater than 70.[143] Median survival with treatment remains less than 1 year.

## Cervical Cancer

Women with HIV experience a higher rate of invasive and preinvasive cervical neoplasia compared with women who are HIV negative. Unlike the incidence of other AIDS-related malignancies, which peaked in the mid 1990s, the incidence of cervical cancer continues to increase.[195] HPV is present in 100% of all cervical cancer cases, but other factors must exist for cervical cancer to develop. While HIV appears to affect the history of HPV infection, and the distribution of genotypes detected in precancerous lesions in HIV-infected women is not similar to that of the general population, the quadrivalent vaccine against HPV appears to be immunogenic in HIV-infected women aged 13 to 45 years with HIV ribonucleic acid levels greater than 10,000 copies/mL and/or CD4 counts greater than 200 cells/mcL.[196,197] In these patients the degree of immunosuppression also can predict the occurrence and severity of cervical disease.[198-200] Cervical malignancy in this population can be aggressive, and screening with cervical cytology can detect disease before it is invasive. Standard screening should be routine, and efforts are underway to integrate cervical cancer screening into HIV care in developing countries.[201] If abnormalities are detected, close follow-up by a provider with experience in HIV-related cervical disease is essential.

## Opportunistic Infections in End-Stage AIDS

Many opportunistic illnesses in end-stage AIDS can be simply and effectively palliated with disease-specific treatments, whereas others are best palliated with nonspecific palliative therapies. A concern is that the treatment of HIV-related cancers may reduce cellular immunity and thus increase the risk of opportunistic infections.[202] Because each patient's response to opportunistic infections and medication side effects is unique, the information in this section should be used only as a guide to treatment. When weighing the burdens and benefits of palliative therapies for opportunistic infections in advanced and end-stage AIDS, clinicians should consider each therapy's effectiveness, ease of administration, side effects, and cost effectiveness. Consultation with an HIV specialist is recommended. The patient's functional status and prognosis should also guide treatment. This approach applies both to primary treatment of infections and to secondary prophylaxis of opportunistic illnesses.[77]

### Pneumocystis Jirovecii Pneumonia

*Pneumocystis carinii* pneumonia, now called *Pneumocystis jirovecii* pneumonia, responds very well to appropriate antimicrobial disease–specific therapy with few side effects. *Pneumocystis* cannot be cultured; the gold-standard in diagnosis is bronchoscopy with bronchoalveolar lavage.[203] Noninvasive diagnostic tests and biomarkers show promise, but these must be validated.[203] Recommended treatments are quite cost effective. It is less burdensome and less expensive to palliate the persistent cough, dyspnea, and fever of *P jirovecii* with trimethoprim-sulfamethoxazole than to treat each symptom individually with multiple palliative agents, although an emerging concern with the use of trimethoprim-sulfamethoxazole is a putative resistance to the drug.[203] In the final stages of a patient's life, *P jirovecii* can be palliated with prednisone, which may also increase the patient's appetite and sense of well-being.

### Toxoplasmosis

Prior to ART, toxoplasmosis was the most common focal cerebral lesion detected in AIDS patients with toxoplasma infection, occurring in approximately half of toxoplasma-seropositive patients. Other forms of dissemination also have been reported in AIDS patients in sites such as the eyes, lungs, heart, and spinal cord. Antitoxoplasma therapy and chemoprophylaxis have shown effectiveness in reducing the incidence of toxoplasmosis, while noncompliance has been identified as a cause of relapse in these settings. Toxoplasmosis is one of the most common neuropathological complications found at autopsy. Rapid progress in the development of ART has changed the observed patterns with this complication, for which there has been a marked decrease in overall incidence. Subsequently, toxoplasmosis has been found to be significantly associated with the so-called neurological immune restoration inflammatory syndrome (NIRIS).[204]

Toxoplasmosis usually presents with seizures, focal neurological deficits, fever, and possibly headache. Positron emission tomography-computed tomography (PET-CT) scans can differentiate between the cerebral lesions of lymphoma and toxoplasmosis in patients with AIDS; such differentiation cannot reliably be achieved with either CT or MRI alone.[205] The current recommended disease-specific treatment for toxoplasmosis is the most effective palliative intervention. Toxoplasmosis should be comanaged with an infectious disease specialist when possible.

### Cryptococcal Meningitis

Cryptococcosis is a systemic infection caused by *Cryptococcus neoformans*. Cryptococcal meningitis can occur in patients with late-stage HIV infection and other types of immunosuppressive disease.[206] Although ART improves survival in persons with cryptococcal meningitis and AIDS, ART frequently elicits HIV immune reconstitution inflammatory syndrome, an exaggerated and frequently deadly inflammatory reaction that complicates recovery from immunodeficiency. Mortality can exceed 30%.[207] ART should not be initiated in patients with cryptococcal meningitis until they have recovered sufficiently.[208] Severe headaches from increased intracranial pressure are common. The amount of opioid analgesia necessary to treat the unremitting headaches of cryptococcal meningitis would cause deep sleep in most people. Treatment with amphotericin, followed by an azole antifungal agent, clearly is preferable. Like *P jirovecii,* toxoplasmosis and cryptococcosis may be palliated with corticosteroids in the final stages of life, which also would reduce the chronic nausea associated with increased intracranial pressure. Serial lumbar puncture is another useful strategy to relieve intracranial pressure and resulting symptoms.

## Mycobacterium Avium Complex

Disseminated MAC infection is a late complication of AIDS. Its manifestations are fever, anemia, diarrhea, and weight loss. Often it can be prevented by continuing prophylaxis with azithromycin, 1,200 mg by mouth every week, or clarithromycin, 500 mg by mouth twice daily. If MAC develops while a patient is in hospice, it can be palliated with antipyretics and antidiarrheals. A course of disease-specific palliative antimicrobial therapy also may be reasonable.

## Cytomegalovirus Enteropathy or Neuropathy

Managing CMV retinitis is a persistent challenge for hospice and palliative medicine physicians. Preservation of sight is the focus, but treatment is invasive, expensive, and laden with potentially major side effects. Current therapy involves initial induction treatment with intravenous agents such as ganciclovir or foscarnet followed by placement of intraocular antimicrobial reservoirs and maintenance oral therapy with ganciclovir or valganciclovir. Individuals with known or suspected CMV should be referred for an ophthalmologic evaluation and initial treatment before admission to a hospice program.

The best treatment for certain opportunistic infections, such as CMV enteropathy or neuropathy, may be typical palliative therapies. Patients in the final stages of life may not experience rapid disease progression before death and therefore may not require disease-specific treatment. Serious toxicities, difficulties with administration of medication, the need for frequent laboratory monitoring, and high cost argue against CMV therapy in all but the most extreme cases.

The CDC's latest prophylaxis recommendations for opportunistic infections[209,210] and other resources are available at http://aidsinfo.nih.gov/contentfiles/lvguidelines/adult_oi.pdf (accessed January 5, 2017).

## *Viral Hepatitis*

Coinfection with hepatitis C virus (HCV) and HIV is common. In the United States the prevalence of HCV is estimated at 1.8%, but the prevalence in individuals who are HIV positive has been reported to range from 12% to 90%.[211,212] A 1999 study estimated that 30%

of individuals who are HIV positive are coinfected with HCV.[213] HCV infection is strongly correlated with the use of illegal drugs (especially injected drugs) and unsafe sexual practices in both HIV-positive and HIV-negative populations, particularly in men who have sex with men.[214] The probability of progression to death or a new AIDS-defining clinical event is independently associated with HCV seropositivity.[215] The rate of progression to cirrhosis for patients coinfected with HCV and HIV is three times higher than the rate for patients only infected with HCV.[216,217] This accelerated rate is magnified in those with low CD4 cell counts. Consumption of alcoholic beverages can also hasten the progression of cirrhosis in people infected with HCV.[218] HCV coinfection also complicates HIV treatment because of the increased frequency of ART-related hepatotoxicity.

Coinfection with HIV and hepatitis B has been reported in approximately 9% of people with HIV.[219] Coinfection with hepatitis A or B increases progression of cirrhosis in HCV-infected individuals. No data demonstrate that the treatment of hepatitis B improves the course of HIV. However, flares of hepatitis-B activity can result in liver-associated toxicities, which in turn can have an impact on the treatment of coinfected individuals. Cirrhosis and end-stage liver disease are increasingly common causes of death for individuals who have HIV.[220] This is particularly true for people receiving ART, for whom AIDS-defining illness and AIDS-related deaths have become much less common.[221]

Historically, treating HCV with pegylated interferon (PEG-INF) and ribavirin has produced sustained viral response rates above 80% for patients without HIV and 46% in HIV-coinfected patients with favorable genotypes.[222,223] This treatment appears to have antiatherogenic effects in patients with and without HIV infection,[224] yet treatment rates, especially in urban centers, remain low.[225,226] Interferon and ribavirin are associated with many side effects; their use is contraindicated for those with mild or advanced cirrhosis, active substance abuse, and depression. Newer agents, such as the combined formulation of ledipasvir and sofosbuvir, appear to be promising in the HIV-infected population. However, given the complicated pharmacological interactions of these agents with ART, providers with expertise in HCV and HIV should be consulted. Liver transplantation is no longer considered a contraindication for end-stage liver disease in coinfected patients; however, the 5-year survival rate for coinfected patients is lower than it is for patients with only HCV (33% vs 72%, $P = .07$).[227] After end-stage cirrhosis and liver failure develop, treatment becomes purely palliative because no disease-specific treatment exists for either condition. The mainstays of palliative treatment are judicious use of diuretics, including furosemide and spironolactone to control edema, and vitamin K to partially reverse coagulopathy.

Prevention of progression to end-stage cirrhosis should be a priority for all clinicians caring for individuals with HIV. HCV is a sexually transmitted blood-borne disease. Individuals without HCV who continue injecting illicit drugs should be counseled to use a sterile needle and syringe for every injection. HCV-infected individuals should be strongly counseled to accept treatment and to not drink alcohol, because it hastens the progression to cirrhosis and liver failure. Individuals with HCV infection who are hepatitis A and B negative should be vaccinated against these viruses because coinfection will speed the progression of cirrhosis and liver failure.

## Clinical Situation

### Juan's Case Concludes (continued from page 17)

You determine Juan is eligible for hospice care with a primary diagnosis of lung cancer. You prescribe nortriptyline 25 mg orally before bedtime and, even though Juan now is in hospice, you continue ART because his HIV infection has responded appropriately to therapy and he may still derive some benefit from continued HIV treatment.

Juan's pain improves over the next 10 days. Juan's children and siblings are visiting him, and even though his cancer is clearly progressing, he is experiencing a peaceful life transition.

After 2 months Juan begins to experience a rather rapid downhill course. He is losing weight despite using dronabinol and megestrol. He is weaker, coughing frequently, and short of breath at rest. He needs help with all his activities of daily living (ADLs) and can no longer leave the house. He has little or no appetite.

Juan has entered the final phase of his life, and ART can no longer provide him with any comfort or prevent any HIV-related illnesses. His ART is discontinued. Juan and his family are likely to benefit from increased home visits by the hospice team, in particular the hospice nurse, home health aides, and the chaplain. Like many people at the end of life, Juan may wish to talk with clergy or other people about spiritual, religious, or existential issues of meaning. Eating less or not eating at all are normal parts of the dying process, and artificial nutrition and aggressive use of appetite stimulants rarely are helpful for individuals who are terminally ill and entering the final phase of their lives. Within a week, Juan dies comfortably, surrounded by his family and friends. His family receives follow-up bereavement care from the hospice program for a year.

 ART may be continued in hospice until the benefits of continued therapy are outweighed by the burdens of treatment (eg, pill burden, adverse effects, medication interactions). If the HIV/AIDS is not contributing to the patient's terminal prognosis, medications can be obtained outside of the benefit. However, access to ART may be challenging when a patient is enrolled in hospice care due to the costs of obtaining or providing ART.

## Discontinuing ART and Opportunitistic Infection Prophylaxes

This section refers to patients with end-stage AIDS as defined in the Prognosis section (see page 4). It does not refer to withdrawing ART from individuals who are clinically stable with detectable HIV viral loads on therapy; such individuals are not generally considered to be hospice candidates unless they have other end-stage comorbidities.

ART works by blocking the replication of HIV. When therapy is successful, the patient's HIV viral load becomes undetectable or decreases markedly from baseline. The patient's immune status recovers, as evidenced by an increase in or stabilization of CD4 lymphocytes. When ART is unsuccessful, patients experience uncontrolled viral replication; progressive loss of CD4 lymphocytes; progression of opportunistic diseases (eg, thrush, MAC, CMV, PML); and a variety of systemic conditions, including seborrheic dermatitis, weight loss, fevers, and fatigue. Continuing unsuccessful ART for patients with end-stage AIDS provides no medical benefit. In fact, ART may do harm because the side effects of ART often worsen when patients reach the end of life.[228]

One of the most difficult decisions faced by patients, families, and healthcare professionals is withdrawing ART and prophylaxis of opportunistic infections. Unfortunately no comprehensive guidelines have been published that address the appropriate time to withdraw ART for patients who have no realistic possibility of benefit.[229] A decision to discontinue ART should be based on the patient's goals of care, the treatment's demonstrated lack of effectiveness, and the treatment's potential to do harm if continued. A decision to withdraw prophylaxis for opportunistic infections should be based on the patient's goals, prognosis, and the burden of continuing this therapy. In the final weeks of life, prophylaxis provides only theoretical benefit.

Patients and family members may resist withdrawing ART because of fears that discontinuation means the situation is hopeless and the patient will die. Even when ART is clearly providing no objective medical benefit, patients and families can find comfort in its continued use. Clinicians also may resist discontinuing ineffective ART because of their own grief over the impending death of a patient for whom they feel great affection. They may be unable to hear a patient's own wishes to discontinue ART.

When people who are infected with HIV and are on successful ART develop a fatal illness secondary to cirrhosis, cancer, coronary artery disease, or other comorbid or unrelated conditions, they may choose to continue ART because it offers benefits such as improved immune function and overall well-being.

An essential element of resolving conflicts in the context of an ongoing relationship is to initially build on areas of trust and consensus when they exist before addressing areas of greatest contention. Eliciting patients' and families' beliefs about the benefits and burdens of continuing ART and their concerns about end-of-life care can be valuable for everyone. Providing consistent information about the burdens and benefits of continuing ART is important.

Patients and family members also should understand that discontinuing ineffective ART may not lead to a rapid worsening of the patient's clinical status; the patient may experience a significant period of well-being after ART is discontinued. When information is shared truthfully and compassionately in the context of a trusting patient-clinician relationship, patients and family members may be willing to discontinue ineffective therapies (see *UNIPAC 5*).

See **Table 8** for potential benefits and risks of ART in late-stage HIV disease.[36]

## Discontinuing Antibiotic Therapy

Formerly beneficial treatments may need to be modified during the last stages of a patient's life. Decisions to discontinue antibiotics should be based on the patient's prognosis and the treatment's likely burdens and benefits from the patient's point of view. For example, prophylactic antibiotic therapies could be discontinued in the last 3 to 4 weeks of life but resumed if the patient becomes symptomatic. Fever-suppressant therapy or short courses of antibiotics may be used to control symptoms such as the fevers and sweats secondary to MAC. When a patient is resistant to oral antifungal medications, a brief course of intravenous therapy may be beneficial if it offers rapid relief of distressing symptoms. Diagnostic procedures and prolonged courses of therapy during the last weeks of a patient's life are likely to pose significant burdens with few benefits.

### Table 8. Potential Benefits and Risks of ART in Late-Stage HIV Disease[36]

| Potential Benefits* | Potential Risks |
|---|---|
| Selection of "less fit" virus (ie, less pathogenic than wild-type virus), even in the presence of elevated viral loads | Cumulative and multiple drug toxicities in the setting of therapeutic futility |
| Protection against HIV encephalopathy and dementia[230] | Diminished QOL from demands of treatment regimen |
| Relief or easing of symptoms possibly associated with high viral loads (eg, constitutional symptoms)* | Therapeutic confusion (ie, use of future-directed, disease-modifying therapy in a dying patient) |
| Continued therapeutic effect, albeit attenuated | Distraction from end-of-life and advance care planning issues, with narrow focus on medication adherence and monitoring |
| Psychological and emotional benefits of continued "disease-combating" therapy | |

*Evidence is lacking for some of these potential benefits, although they are commonly considered in clinical decision making.*

## Conversations Near the End of Life

Families and healthcare professionals may fear that discussing death will frighten the person who is dying or cause a loss of hope, but this is not the case in most situations. Most people know when they are dying and are relieved when they can discuss their hopes and fears with caring family members, friends, and healthcare professionals. Some people may feel a need to protect others by avoiding discussions of death-related topics, especially with their family members. They may be more comfortable talking about their impending death with healthcare professionals and friends.

As they are dying, most people want to know that their time on Earth has been worthwhile, that they have been loved and will be remembered, and that they have been forgiven for past transgressions. Such conversations are particularly important for people dying from HIV/AIDS because of the stigma attached to the disease. Participating in a life review gives patients an opportunity to recognize important themes in their lives and can provide reassurance that they will live on in the memories of family and friends.

Family members and friends may say goodbye and give the dying patient permission to go. Permission to die also may be granted verbally by healthcare professionals who have become friends with the patient during the course of a long illness.

Saying "goodbye" may be the most difficult conversation for both the dying person and those who will be left behind because it acknowledges the finality of life. People who are dying also must be reassured that their loved ones will be able to care for themselves after the death occurs. This is especially important for those who have served as caregivers for spouses and children. Reassurance is vital when survivors include young children.

See *UNIPAC 5* for more information on communicating with patients and family members.

## Grief and Multiple Losses

HIV has caused the deaths of millions of people. Because the virus most often spreads through intimate contact, several friends and acquaintances may be sick or dying at the same time. Grieving the anticipated or actual death of one friend is always stressful; grieving the deaths of many in succession can overwhelm a survivor's coping mechanisms and even accelerate his or her own HIV disease.[231]

Some people with HIV disease have experienced the deaths of several friends and family members over a period of years. The same holds true for healthcare professionals who treat patients with HIV disease. We are only beginning to learn how to help people cope with the multiple losses associated with AIDS.[232] The traditional bereavement model may be inadequate for survivors of multiple AIDS-related deaths. Members of the gay community, for example, often receive little support when trying to cope with their grief. Qualitative research on same-sex couples who are grieving has revealed several common themes, among them "tacit acknowledgment," "sculpting the distress," "multiple losses," "seeking support," and "journeying anew."[233] Those who experience multiple deaths often experience the loss of the people they ordinarily go to for support.[234] In addition, bereavement in the lesbian, gay, bisexual, and transgender (LGBT) community can be complicated by factors such as the failure to acknowledge the relationship, legal and financial issues, and stigma of HIV/AIDS.[235]

Just as Elisabeth Kübler-Ross described stages in patients' reactions to dying, David Nord has described four stages of responding to multiple AIDS-related deaths.[236] These stages are not exclusive and may occur randomly or contemporaneously:

- shock and denial
- overload and confusion
- facing of reality
- reinvestment and recovery.

Grieving involves a process of adjusting to an irrevocable loss of objects, relationships, and dreams. According to Nord, social support, community involvement, and a sense of purpose can help survivors achieve a sense of empowerment and reduce their sense of victimization.[236]

Healthcare professionals can use the following strategies to help survivors negotiate the grieving process:

- Normalize feelings of grief.
- Provide education about common reactions to loss so survivors won't believe they are "going crazy."
- Reassure grieving people that they, as survivors, will be able to live with their grief and that help is available, if needed.

Coping-focused interventions have demonstrated some effectiveness.[237] Achieving a sense of balance in life and pursuing a life despite AIDS can help survivors develop a necessary sense of detachment. Physical exercise, meditation, and vacations away from usual environments are effective means of preventing and responding to burnout. An active sense of humor is also helpful.

*Bearing witness* refers to keeping the dead person's memory alive.[236] The AIDS quilt project is a good example of such a witness, demonstrating the power and importance of ritual. Making a quilt panel is a shared experience that offers support for the makers of the quilt and for viewers.

Holding memorial services on a regular basis can be comforting and can help give survivors a sense of closure. Survivors of multiple losses may be afraid to openly grieve for fear they will be unable to maintain or regain control or ever stop crying. Holding onto grief produces a syndrome similar to that seen with burnout. Symptoms include emotional numbing, withdrawal from others, misdirected anger, lack of pleasure in anything, and resorting to drugs or alcohol to cope with everyday life.[238] See *UNIPAC 2* for further information on alleviating psychological and spiritual pain and grief and bereavement. See *UNIPAC 5* for more information on communicating with patients and families and coping with stress and burnout.

# Issues for Caregivers

## Stress and Burnout

Occupational stress and burnout commonly affect health professionals who care for patients with chronic illnesses such as cancer or HIV/AIDS.[239] The care of patients with HIV/AIDS has become increasingly complex with the advent of ART because patients are living longer. Decisions related to withdrawal of care, goals of therapy, and acceptance of treatment failure and death in the age of ART are different from those in the previous era, during which the death of these patients was expected, imminent, and universal. The possibility of success from the next regimen or the next new drug complicates these issues from the providers' and patients' perspectives. Nurses working with patients who are HIV positive may suffer burnout sooner than those caring for patients with cancer. Staff turnover, absenteeism, and reduced productivity are symptoms of burnout.

Coping style is associated with burnout. People with an *external* coping style believe that the locus of control exists outside the individual, that they have no control over circumstances and must simply accept what is happening. Such caregivers tend to exhibit a fatalistic attitude and use denial as a coping mechanism, which is an ineffective strategy for resolving grief. People with an *internal* coping style believe that the locus of control exists within each individual. They are more likely to express their emotions and use healthy strategies for relieving stress—for example, by taking vacations and engaging in physical exercise. Individuals with an internal coping style generally feel more in control of their own fate.

The dichotomy between external and internal coping styles has been noted in healthcare providers. The age of the caregiver and the heaviness of the care load, although independent predictors of burnout, does not outweigh the influence of locus of control. Healthcare professionals can learn to use appropriate coping mechanisms tailored to their situation. Hospice and palliative medicine physicians have reported a number of coping strategies to avoid burnout.[240] The most common strategy reported was attending to physical well-being (60%), followed by maintaining professional relationships (57%), taking a transcendental perspective (43%), talking with others (43%), engaging in hobbies (40%), ensuring variety in clinical practice (37%), maintaining personal relationships (37%), and observing personal boundaries (37%). Having "time away" from work (27%), sustaining passion for one's work (20%), having realistic expectations (13%), using humor and laughter (13%), and remembering patients (10%) were cited less frequently.[240]

## Sexual Exposure to HIV and Preexposure Prophylaxis

The prevention of HIV transmission during sexual contact is important at any trajectory of HIV disease, including those near the end of life and their sexual contacts. In 2012 the US Food and Drug Administration approved the use of a fixed-dose combination of tenofovir disoproxil fumarate and emtricitabine to reduce the risk of sexually acquired HIV. This approval was in addition to the standard use of barrier protection (eg, condoms) and screening and counseling for sexually transmitted infections. It also was based on several clinical trials that demonstrated a substantial reduction in the rate of transmission of HIV in men who have sex with men, discordant heterosexual couples, and others at risk for sexual acquisition of HIV.[241] In 2014 the US Public Health Service published a clinical practice guideline for the use of preexposure prophylaxis (PREP) to prevent HIV transmission in the United States.[242]

### Occupational Exposure to HIV

The CDC gathers information about healthcare worker exposure to HIV. As of December 31, 2013, 58 confirmed occupational transmissions of HIV and 150 possible transmissions had been reported in the United States. Of these, only one confirmed case has been reported since 1999.[243] Risks for seroconversion include deep injury, visible blood on a device, previous needle placement in a vein or artery, and a source with late-stage HIV infection or any patient with a high viral burden.

The CDC guidelines for postexposure evaluation and treatment[244] emphasize the importance of determining the extent of exposure before making a decision about antiretroviral prophylaxis. If exposure occurs, it is advisable to discuss recommended management with an infection control officer in the nearest hospital or, if that person is not available, with the covering physician for infectious diseases. The CDC operates the National Clinicians' Post-Exposure Prophylaxis Hotline at 888.HIV.4911.

## Internet Resources

The care of patients with HIV/AIDS is a dynamic and rapidly changing field. The palliative care of such patients is also changing at a rapid pace. In addition to collaborating with HIV/AIDS experts, palliative medicine physicians should actively use Internet resources in the care of their patients. Reputable sites include the following (all accessible as of August 4, 2017):

- Centers for Disease Control and Prevention, www.cdc.gov/hiv—up-to-date information about epidemiology, prevention, and clinical and public health issues in HIV/AIDS
- World Health Organization, www.who.int/hiv/en—current information about global efforts to treat and prevent HIV/AIDS
- National Institutes of Health, https://aidsinfo.nih.gov—information on HIV/AIDS treatment, prevention, and research, including downloadable tools
- AIDS.ORG, www.aids.org—education and materials facilitating the open exchange of knowledge in accordance with the organization's mission: to help prevent HIV infections and to improve the lives of those affected by HIV/AIDS
- American Academy of HIV Medicine, https://aahivm.org—support for healthcare providers in HIV medicine, including the study guide *AAHIVM Fundamentals of HIV Medicine,* 2007 edition, under the auspices of this independent organization of HIV specialists dedicated to promoting excellence in HIV/AIDS care

- Johns Hopkins HIV Guide, https://www.hopkinsguides.com/hopkins/ub—comprehensive guide to the care of patients with HIV, along with Hopkins AIDS Reports; site requires free registration
- The University of Liverpool, www.hiv-druginteractions.org—comprehensive information on drug interactions and new therapeutics in HIV medicine, sponsored by pharmaceutical companies
- Henry J. Kaiser Family Foundation, http://www.kff.org/hivaids—information on federal spending data, US state HIV/AIDS information, and a daily news service that features HIV/AIDS policy information, webcasts of special events, and public opinion research
- Medscape HIV/AIDS, www.medscape.com/hiv—coverage of major HIV/AIDS conferences, news feeds, online continuing medical education courses, and special feature articles; site requires one-time free registration.

## Future Directions

Once a uniformly fatal illness, HIV/AIDS has rapidly become a chronic illness with episodes of exacerbation and remission, similar to other chronic diseases (eg, heart failure, chronic obstructive pulmonary disease, dementia, renal disease, neurological disorders). With prolonged life expectancy, individuals with HIV/AIDS now face a host of complex medical, psychosocial, and spiritual difficulties. Physicians, other healthcare providers, family members, and caregivers also face new challenges.

Challenges, however, can bring opportunity. Palliative care was built on the principles of relieving suffering through education, research, and interdisciplinary collaboration. If we remain true to these principles, we will continue to improve the care of patients with HIV.

# References

1.  Centers for Disease Control and Prevention, US Department of Health and Human Services. HIV surveillance—United States, 1981-2008. *MMWR Morb Mortal Wkly Rep.* 2011;60(21):689-693.

2.  Centers for Disease Control and Prevention, US Department of Health and Human Services. HIV in the United States: At a Glance. https://www.cdc.gov/hiv/statistics/overview/ataglance.html. Accessed June 27, 2017.

3.  Selwyn PA. Palliative care for patient with human immunodeficiency virus/acquired immune deficiency syndrome. *J Palliat Med.* 2005;8(6):1248-1268.

4.  Centers for Disease Control and Prevention, US Department of Health and Human Services. *HIV Surveillance Report, 2013.* 2015;25. https://www.cdc.gov/hiv/pdf/library/reports/surveillance/cdc-hiv-surveillance-report-2013-vol-25.pdf. Accessed June 27, 2017.

5.  Pitts M, Grierson J, Misson S. Growing older with HIV: a study of health, social and economic circumstances for people living with HIV in Australia over the age of 50 years. *AIDS Patient Care STDS.* 2005;19(7):460-465.

6.  Hooshyar D, Hanson D, Wolfe M, Selik R, Buskin S, McNaghten A. Trends in perimortal conditions and mortality rates among HIV-infected patients. *AIDS.* 2007;21(15):2093-2100.

7.  Palella F, Baker R, Moorman A, et al. Mortality in the highly active antiretroviral therapy era: changing causes of death and disease in the HIV outpatient study. *J Acquir Immune Defic Syndr.* 2006;43(1):27-34.

8.  Simon P, Hu D, Diaz T, Kerndt P. Income and AIDS rates in Los Angeles County. *AIDS.* 1995;9(3):281-284.

9.  Peterman T, Lindsey C, Selik R. This place is killing me: a comparison of counties where the incidence rates of AIDS increased the most and the least. *J Infect Dis.* 2005;191(Suppl 1):S123-S126.

10. McFarland W, Chen S, Hsu L, Schwarcz S, Katz M. Low socioeconomic status is associated with a higher rate of death in the era of highly active antiretroviral therapy. *J Acquir Immune Defic Syndr.* 2003;33(1):96-103.

11. Cunningham W, Hays R, Duan N, et al. The effect of socioeconomic status on the survival of people receiving care for HIV infection in the United States. *J Health Care Poor Underserved.* 2005;16(4):655-676.

12. Krakauer E. Just palliative care: responding responsibly to the suffering of the poor. *J Pain Symptom Manage.* 2008;36(5):505-512.

13. Selwyn P. Palliative care and social justice. *J Pain Symptom Manage.* 2008;36(5):513-515.

14. Cassell EJ. Diagnosing suffering: a perspective. *Ann Intern Med.* 1999;131(7):531-534.

15. O'Neill JF, Alexander CS. Palliative medicine and HIV/AIDS. *Prim Care.* 1997;24(3):607-615.

16. Barroso J. A review of fatigue in people with HIV infection. *J Assoc Nurses AIDS Care.* 1999;10(5):42-49.

17. Webel A. Testing a peer-based symptom intervention for women living with HIV/AIDS. *AIDS Care.* 2010;22(9):1029-1040.

18. Cunningham W, Wong M, Hays R. Case management and health-related quality of life in a national sample of persons with HIV/AIDS. *J Natl Med Assoc.* 2008;100(7):840-847.

19. Farsides C. Allowing someone to die. In: Scherr L, ed. *Grief and AIDS.* New York, NY: John Wiley and Sons; 1995:103-112.

20. Breitbart W, Rosenfeld BD, Passik SD, McDonald MV, Thaler H, Portenoy RK. The undertreatment of pain in ambulatory AIDS patients. *Pain.* 1996;65(2-3):243-249.

21. Sowell RL, Seals BF, Moneyham L, Demi A, Cohen L, Brake S. Quality of life in HIV-infected women in the southeastern United States. *AIDS Care.* 1997;9(5):501-512.

22. Cook JA, Grey D, Burke J, et al. Depressive symptoms and AIDS-related mortality among a multisite cohort of HIV-positive women. *Am J Public Health.* 2004;94(7):1133-1140.

23. Siegel K, Karus D, Dean L. Psychosocial characteristics of New York City HIV-infected women before and after the advent of HAART. *Am J Public Health*. 2004;94(7):1127-1132.

24. Cederfjall C, Langius-Eklof A, Lidman K, Wredling R. Gender differences in perceived health-related quality of life among patients with HIV infection. *AIDS Patient Care STDS*. 2001;15(1):31-39.

25. Cook JA, Cohen MH, Burke J, et al. Effects of depressive symptoms and mental health quality of life on use of highly active antiretroviral therapy among HIV-seropositive women. *J Acquir Immune Defic Syndr*. 2002;30(4):401-409.

26. te Vaarwerk MJ, Gaal EA. Psychological distress and quality of life in drug-using and non-drug-using HIV-infected women. *Eur J Public Health*. 2001;11(1):109-115.

27. Wingwood G, Diclemente R, Mikhail I, et al. HIV discrimination and the health of women living with HIV. *Womens Health*. 2007;46(2-3):99-112.

28. Andrinopoulos K, Clum G, Murphy DA, et al. Health related quality of life and psychosocial correlates among HIV-infected adolescent and young adult women in the US. *AIDS Educ Prev*. 2011;23(4):367-381.

29. Hader SL, Smith DK, Moore JS, Holmberg SD. HIV infection in women in the United States: status at the Millennium. *JAMA*. 2001;285(9):1186-1192.

30. Moore J, Schuman P, Schoenbaum E, Boland B, Solomon L, Smith D. Severe adverse life events and depressive symptoms among women with, or at risk for, HIV infection in four cities in the United States of America. *AIDS*. 1999;13(17):2459-2468.

31. Eastwood EA, Fletcher J, Quinlivan EB, Verdecias N, Birnbaum JM, Blank AE. Baseline social characteristics and barriers to care from a Special Projects of National Significance Women of Color with HIV study: a comparison of urban and rural women and barriers to HIV care. *AIDS Patient Care STDS*. 2015;29 Suppl 1:S4-10.

32. Altice F, Kamarulzaman A, Soriano V, Schecter M, Friedland G. Treatment of medical, psychiatric and substance-use comorbidities in people infected with HIV, who use drugs. *Lancet*. 2010;376(9738):367-387.

33. Chatterjee K. Host genetic factors in susceptibility to HIV-1 infection and progression to AIDS. *J Genet*. 2010;89(1):109-116.

34. Selwyn PA, Rivard M. Palliative care for AIDS: challenges and opportunities in the era of highly active anti-retroviral therapy. *J Palliat Med*. 2003;6(3):475-487.

35. Oppenheim S. Fast Facts and Concepts #213: Prognosis in HIV and AIDS. 2009; https://www.mypcnow.org/blank-uh2m9. Accessed June 27, 2017.

36. Selwyn PA, Forstein M. Overcoming the false dichotomy of curative vs palliative care for late-stage HIV/AIDS: "let me live the way I want to live, until I can't". *JAMA*. 2003;290(6):806-814.

37. Bhaskaran K, Hamouda O, Sannes M, et al. Changes in the risk of death after HIV seroconversion compared with mortality in the general population. *JAMA*. 2008;300(1):51-59.

38. Krentz H, Kliewer G, Gill M. Changing mortality rates and causes of death for HIV-infected individuals living in Southern Alberta, Canada, from 1998 to 2003. *HIV Med*. 2005;6(2):99-106.

39. Quinlivan EB, Fletcher J, Eastwood EA, Blank AE, Verdecias N, Roytburd K. Health status of HIV-infected women entering care: baseline medical findings from the women of color initiative. *AIDS Patient Care STDS*. 2015;29 Suppl 1:S11-19.

40. Antiretroviral Therapy Cohort Collaboration, University of Bristol. Risk calculators. www.bristol.ac.uk/art-cc/research/calculator/. Accessed June 27, 2017.

41. May M, Sterne JA, Sabin C, et al. Prognosis of HIV-1-infected patients up to 5 years after initiation of HAART: collaborative analysis of prospective studies. *AIDS*. 2007;21(9):1185-1197.

42. Anastos K, Barron Y, Cohen MH, et al. The prognostic importance of changes in CD4+ cell count and HIV-1 RNA level in women after initiating highly active antiretroviral therapy. *Ann Intern Med*. 2004;140(4):256-264.

43. Reiter G, Gardner E, Wojtusik L, Wojnarowski C. HAART treatment yields no AIDS death in an inner-city population over three years. Paper presented at: DART 2000, Frontiers in Drug Development for Antiretroviral Therapy; December 17-21, 2000; San Juan, PR.

44. Reiter G, Stewart K, Wojtusik L, et al. Elements of success in HIV clinical care—multiple interventions that promote adherence. *Topics HIV Med*. 2000;8(5):21-30.

45. Srasuebkul P, Lim P, Lee M, et al. Short-term clinical disease progression in HIV-infected patients receiving combination antiretroviral therapy: results from the TREAT Asia HIV observational database. *Clin Infect Dis*. 2009;48(7):940-950.

46. Carrico A, Riley E, Johnson M, et al. Psychiatric risk factors for HIV disease progression: the role of inconsistent patterns of antiretroviral therapy utilization. *J Acquir Immune Defic Syndr*. 2011;56(2):145-150.

47. Zolopa AR, Hahn JA, Gorter R, et al. HIV and tuberculosis infection in San Francisco's homeless adults. Prevalence and risk factors in a representative sample. *JAMA*. 1994;272(6):455-461.

48. Nelson EC, Stason WB, Neutra RR, Solomon HS. Identification of the noncompliant hypertensive patient. *Prev Med*. 1980;9(4):504-517.

49. Stanton AL. Determinants of adherence to medical regimens by hypertensive patients. *J Behav Med*. 1987;10(4):377-394.

50. DeVon HA, Powers MJ. Health beliefs, adjustment to illness, and control of hypertension. *Res Nurs Health*. 1984;7(1):10-16.

51. Samet JH, Libman H, Steger KA, et al. Compliance with zidovudine therapy in patients infected with human immunodeficiency virus, type 1: a cross-sectional study in a municipal hospital clinic. *Am J Med*. 1992;92(5):495-502.

52. Rao D, Kekwaletswe TC, Hosek S, Martinez J, Rodriguez F. Stigma and social barriers to medication adherence with urban youth living with HIV. *AIDS Care*. 2007;19(1):28-33.

53. Mack JW, Block SD, Nilsson M, et al. Measuring therapeutic alliance between oncologists and patients with advanced cancer: the Human Connection Scale. *Cancer*. 2009;115(14):3302-3311.

54. Davison SN, Simpson C. Hope and advance care planning in patients with end stage renal disease: qualitative interview study. *BMJ*. 2006;333(7574):886.

55. Bennett L. AIDS health care: staff stress, loss and bereavement. In: Scherr L, ed. *Grief and AIDS*. New York, NY: John Wiley and Sons; 1995:87-102.

56. Erlandson KM, Allshouse AA, Duong S, MaWhinney S, Kohrt WM, Campbell TB. HIV, aging, and advance care planning: are we successfully planning for the future? *J Palliat Med*. 2012;15(10):1124-1129.

57. Johnson KS, Elbert-Avila KI, Tulsky JA. The influence of spiritual beliefs and practices on the treatment preferences of African Americans: a review of the literature. *J Am Geriatr Soc*. 2005;53(4):711-719.

58. Voorhees J, Rietjens J, Onwuteaka-Philipsen B, et al. Discussing prognosis with terminally ill cancer patients and relatives: a survey of physicians' intentions in seven countries. *Patient Educ Couns*. 2009;77(3):430-436.

59. Centers for Medicare and Medicaid Services, US Department of Health and Human Services. Local Coverage Determinations (LCDs) by Contractor Index. https://www.cms.gov/medicare-coverage-database/indexes/lcd-contractor-index.aspx. Accessed June 27, 2017.

60. Deeks SG, Hecht FM, Swanson M, et al. HIV RNA and CD4 cell count response to protease inhibitor therapy in an urban AIDS clinic: response to both initial and salvage therapy. *AIDS*. 1999;13(6):F35-43.

61. Valdez H, Lederman MM, Woolley I, et al. Human immunodeficiency virus 1 protease inhibitors in clinical practice: predictors of virological outcome. *Arch Intern Med.* 1999;159(15):1771-1776.

62. Havlir DV, Hellmann NS, Petropoulos CJ, et al. Drug susceptibility in HIV infection after viral rebound in patients receiving indinavir-containing regimens. *JAMA.* 2000;283(2):229-234.

63. Descamps D, Flandre P, Calvez V, et al. Mechanisms of virologic failure in previously untreated HIV-infected patients from a trial of induction-maintenance therapy. Trilege (Agence Nationale de Recherches sur le SIDA 072) Study Team. *JAMA.* 2000;283(2):205-211.

64. Bangsberg DR, Hecht FM, Charlebois ED, et al. Adherence to protease inhibitors, HIV-1 viral load, and development of drug resistance in an indigent population. *AIDS.* 2000;14(4):357-366.

65. Staszewski S, DeMasi R, Hill AM, Dawson D. HIV-1 RNA, CD4 cell count and the risk of progression to AIDS and death during treatment with HIV-1 reverse transcriptase inhibitors. *AIDS.* 1998;12(15):1991-1997.

66. Reiter GS. Clinical correlates of human immunodeficiency virus (HIV)-related immunosuppression. *Semin Ultrasound CT MR.* 1998;19(2):128-132.

67. Buchbinder SP, Holmberg SD, Scheer S, Colfax G, O'Malley P, Vittinghoff E. Combination antiretroviral therapy and incidence of AIDS-related malignancies. *J Acquir Immune Defic Syndr.* 1999;21(Suppl 1):S23-26.

68. Jones JL, Hanson DL, Dworkin MS, Ward JW, Jaffe HW. Effect of antiretroviral therapy on recent trends in selected cancers among HIV-infected persons. Adult/Adolescent Spectrum of HIV Disease Project Group. *J Acquir Immune Defic Syndr.* 1999;21(Suppl 1):S11-17.

69. Aviles A, Halabe J. Improved prognosis in patients with acquired immunodeficiency syndrome-related lymphoma. *Cancer Biother Radiopharm.* 1999;14(5):349-352.

70. Levine AM. Acquired immunodeficiency syndrome-related lymphoma: clinical aspects. *Semin Oncol.* 2000;27(4):442-453.

71. Olszewski AJ, Castillo JJ. Outcomes of HIV-associated Hodgkin lymphoma in the era of antiretroviral therapy. *AIDS.* 2016;30(5):787-796.

72. Bartlett JG. *Medical Management of HIV Infection 2007.* Baltimore, MD: Port City Press; 2007.

73. Panel on Antiretroviral Guidelines for Adults and Adolescents. Guidelines for the Use of Antiretroviral Agents in HIV-1-Infected Adults and Adolescents: US Department of Health and Human Services. www.aidsinfo.nih.gov/ContentFiles/AdultandAdolescentGL.pdf. Accessed June 27, 2017.

74. Szarfman A, DuMouchel W, Fram D, et al. Lactic Acidosis: Unraveling the Individual Toxicities of Drugs Used in HIV and Diabetes Polytherapy by Hierarchical Bayesian Logistic Regression Data Mining. FDA Science Forum; April 27-28, 2005; Washington, DC. https://www.accessdata.fda.gov/ScienceForums/forum05/H-30.htm. Accessed June 27, 2017.

75. Matthews LT, Giddy J, Ghebremichael M, et al. A risk-factor guided approach to reducing lactic acidosis and hyperlactatemia in patients on antiretroviral therapy. *PLoS One.* 2011;6(4):e18736.

76. Cote HC, Brumme ZL, Craib KJ, et al. Changes in mitochondrial DNA as a marker of nucleoside toxicity in HIV-infected patients. *N Engl J Med.* 2002;346(11):811-820.

77. Reiter GS, Kudler NR. Palliative care and HIV, part I: OIs and cancers. *AIDS Clin Care.* 1996;8(3):21-22, 26.

78. Reiter GS, Kudler NR. Palliative care and HIV, part II: systemic manifestations and late-stage issues. *AIDS Clin Care.* 1996;8(4):27-30, 33, 36.

79. Rey D, Partisani M, Krantz V, et al. Prednisolone does not prevent the occurrence of nevirapine-induced rashes. *AIDS.* 1999;13(16):2307.

80. Clarke S, Harrington P, Condon C, Kelleher D, Smith OP, Mulcahy F. Late onset hepatitis and prolonged deterioration in hepatic function associated with nevirapine therapy. *Int J STD AIDS.* 2000;11(5):336-337.

81. Carr A, Samaras K, Chisholm DJ, Cooper DA. Pathogenesis of HIV-1-protease inhibitor-associated peripheral lipodystrophy, hyperlipidaemia, and insulin resistance. *Lancet.* 1998;351(9119):1881-1883.

82. Duong M, Petit J, Piroth L, et al. Lipid evaluation and glucose metabolism in HIV-infected patients before and after initiation of protease inhibitor therapy [abstract]. *Abstr Intersci Conf Antimicrob Agents Chemother.* 1999;39:495. Abstract 1291.

83. Polo R, Verdejo J, Gonzalez-Munoz M, et al. Lipodystrophy related to NRT inhibitors in HAART therapy [abstract]. *Abstr Intersci Conf Antimicrob Agents Chemother.* 1999;39:501. Abstract 1302.

84. Romeu J, Sirerre G, Rego M, et al. Cumulative risk for developing hyperlipidemia in HIV-infected patients treated with protease inhibitors [abstract]. *Abstr Intersci Conf Antimicrob Agents Chemother.* 1999;39:498. Abstract 1293.

85. Ward D, Delaney K, Moorman A, et al. Clinical features related to lipodystrophy severity in the HIV outpatient study [abstract]. *Abstr Intersci Conf Antimicrob Agents Chemother.* 1999:Sept 26-29. Abstract 1299.

86. Mallal S, John M, Moore C, James I, McKinnon E. Protease inhibitors and nucleoside reverse transcriptase inhibitors interact to cause subcutaneous fat wasting in patients with HIV infection [abstract]. *Antivir Ther.* 1999;4(suppl 2):42. Abstract 19.

87. Worm SW, De Wit S, Weber R, et al. Diabetes mellitus, preexisting coronary heart disease, and the risk of subsequent coronary heart disease events in patients infected with human immunodeficiency virus: the Data Collection on Adverse Events of Anti-HIV Drugs (D:A:D Study). *Circulation.* 2009;119(6):805-811.

88. Kilby JM, Tabereaux PB. Severe hyperglycemia in an HIV clinic: preexisting versus drug-associated diabetes mellitus. *J Acquir Immune Defic Syndr Hum Retrovirol.* 1998;17(1):46-50.

89. Vyas AK, Koster JC, Tzekov A, Hruz PW. Effects of the HIV protease inhibitor ritonavir on GLUT4 knock-out mice. *J Biol Chem.* 2010;285(47):36395-36400.

90. Noor MA, Lo JC, Mulligan K, et al. Metabolic effects of indinavir in healthy HIV-seronegative men. *AIDS.* 2001;15(7):F11-18.

91. Saunders C. The challenge of terminal care. In: Symington T, Carter R, eds. *Scientific Foundations of Oncology.* London: Heinemann; 1976:673-679.

92. Kutzen HS. Integration of palliative care into primary care for human immunodeficiency virus-infected patients. *Am J Med Sci.* 2004;328(1):37-47.

93. Ferris F, Flannery J, eds. *A Comprehensive Guide for the Care of Persons with HIV Disease.* Toronto, Canada: Mount Sinai Hospital/Casey House Hospice; 1995.

94. Carr D, Addison R. *Pain in HIV/AIDS.* Washington, DC: France-USA Pain Association; 1994.

95. Sims R, Moss V. *Palliative Care for People with AIDS.* 2nd ed. London: Edward Arnold; 1995.

96. Vogl D, Rosenfeld B, Breitbart W, et al. Symptom prevalence, characteristics, and distress in AIDS outpatients. *J Pain Symptom Manage.* 1999;18(4):253-262.

97. Corless I, Bunch E, Kemppainen J, et al. "Fatigue bigtime": fatigue and weakness in HIV disease under-reported and under-treated [abstract]. *Int Conf AIDS.* 2000;13. Abstract ThPeB5235.

98. Perry BA, Westfall AO, Molony E, et al. Characteristics of an ambulatory palliative care clinic for HIV-infected patients. *J Palliat Med.* 2013;16(8):934-937.

99. Simms VM, Higginson IJ, Harding R. What palliative care-related problems do patients experience at HIV diagnosis? A systematic review of the evidence. *J Pain Symptom Manage.* 2011;42(5):734-753.

100. Siegel K, Bradley CJ, Lekas HM. Causal attributions for fatigue among late middle-aged and older adults with HIV infection. *J Pain Symptom Manage.* 2004;28(3):211-224.

101. Breitbart W, Rosenfeld B, Kaim M, Funesti-Esch J. A randomized, double-blind, placebo-controlled trial of psychostimulants for the treatment of fatigue in ambulatory patients with human immunodeficiency virus disease. *Arch Intern Med.* 2001;161(3):411-420.

102. Barroso J. Physiological and psychosocial factors that predict HIV-related fatigue. *AIDS Behav.* 2010;14(6):1415-1427.

103. Jong E, Oudhoff L, Epskamp C, et al. Predictors and treatment strategies of HIV-related fatigue in the combined antiretroviral therapy era. *AIDS*. 2010;24(10):1387-1405.

104. Pence B, Barroso J, Harmon J, Leserman J, Salahuddin N, Hammill B. Chronicity and remission of fatigue in patients with established HIV infection. *AIDS Patient Care STDS*. 2009;23(4):239-244.

105. Leserman J, Barroso J, Pence B, Salahuddin N, Harmon J. Trauma, stressful life events and depression predict HIV-related fatigue. *AIDS Care*. 2008;20(10):1258-1265.

106. Rabkin J. Modafinil treatment for fatigue in HIV/AIDS: a randomized placebo-controlled study. *J Clin Psychiatry*. 2010;71(6):707-715.

107. Rabkin JG, McElhiney MC, Rabkin R. Treatment of HIV-related fatigue with armodafinil: a placebo-controlled randomized trial. *Psychosomatics*. 2011;52(4):328-336.

108. Taylor JK, Pendleton N. Progesterone therapy for the treatment of non-cancer cachexia: a systematic review. *BMJ Support Palliat Care*. 2016;6(3):276-286.

109. Monkemuller K, Lazenby A, Lee D, Loudon R, Wilcox C. Occurrence of gastrointestinal opportunistic disorders in AIDS despite the use of highly active antiretroviral therapy. *Dig Dis Sci*. 2005;50(2):230-234.

110. Connolly G, Hawkins D, Harcourt-Webster J, Parsons P, Husain O, Gazzard B. Oesophageal symptoms, their causes, treatment, and prognosis in patients with the acquired immunodeficiency syndrome. *Gut*. 1989;30(8):1033-1039.

111. Bonacini M, Young T, Laine L. The causes of esophageal symptoms in human immunodeficiency virus infection. A prospective study of 110 patients. *Arch Intern Med*. 1991;151(8):1567-1572.

112. Wilcox C. Short report: time course of clinical response with fluconazole for Candida oesophagitis in patients with AIDS. *Aliment Pharmacol Ther*. 1994;8(3):347.

113. Bhaijee F, Subramony C, Tang SJ, Pepper DJ. Human immunodeficiency virus-associated gastrointestinal disease: common endoscopic biopsy diagnoses. *Patholog Res Int*. 2011;2011:247923.

114. Wilcox C, Straub R, Clark W. Prospective evaluation of oropharyngeal findings in human immunodeficiency virus-infected patients with esophageal ulceration. *Am J Gastroenterol*. 1995;90(11):1938-1941.

115. Nkuize M, De Wit S, Muls V, Arvanitakis M, Buset M. Upper gastrointestinal endoscopic findings in the era of highly active antiretroviral therapy. *HIV Med*. 2010;11(6):412-417.

116. Wilcox C. Evaluation of the HIV-infected patient with odynophagia and dysphagia. *UpToDate*. http://www.uptodate.com/contents/evaluation-of-the-hiv-infected-patient-with-odynophagia-and-dysphagia. Accessed June 27, 2017.

117. Hill A, Balkin A. Risk factors for gastrointestinal adverse events in HIV treated and untreated patients. *AIDS Rev*. 2009;11(1):30-38.

118. Ledergerber B, Egger M, Erard V, et al. AIDS-related opportunistic illnesses occurring after initiation of potent antiretroviral therapy: the Swiss HIV Cohort Study. *JAMA*. 1999;282(23):2220-2226.

119. Call S, Heudebert G, Saag M, Wilcox C. The changing etiology of chronic diarrhea in HIV-infected patients with CD4 cell counts less than 200/mm$^3$. *Am J Gastroenterol*. 2000;95(11):3142-3146.

120. Mayer H, Wanke C. Diagnostic strategies in HIV-infected patients with diarrhea. *AIDS*. 1994;8(12):1639-1648.

121. Feasey NA, Healey P, Gordon MA. Review article: the aetiology, investigation and management of diarrhoea in the HIV-positive patient. *Aliment Pharmacol Ther*. 2011;34(6):587-603.

122. Wilcox C, Wanke C. Evaluation of the HIV-infected patient with diarrhea. *UpToDate*. http://www.uptodate.com/contents/evaluation-of-the-hiv-infected-patient-with-diarrhea. Accessed June 27, 2017.

123. Stoskopf CH, Kim YK, Glover SH. Dual diagnosis: HIV and mental illness, a population-based study. *Community Ment Health J*. 2001;37(6):469-479.

124. Himelhoch S, Moore RD, Treisman G, Gebo KA. Does the presence of a current psychiatric disorder in AIDS patients affect the initiation of antiretroviral treatment and duration of therapy? *J Acquir Immune Defic Syndr.* 2004;37(4):1457-1463.

125. Sherbourne CD, Hays RD, Fleishman JA, et al. Impact of psychiatric conditions on health-related quality of life in persons with HIV infection. *Am J Psychiatry.* 2000;157(2):248-254.

126. Anderson EH. Self-esteem and optimism in men and women infected with HIV. *Nurs Res.* 2000;49(5):262-271.

127. Moneyham L, Sowell R, Seals B, Demi A. Depressive symptoms among African American women with HIV disease. *Sch Inq Nurs Pract.* 2000;14(1):9-39; discussion 41-36.

128. Goulet JL, Molde S, Constantino J, Gaughan D, Selwyn PA. Psychiatric comorbidity and the long-term care of people with AIDS. *J Urban Health.* 2000;77(2):213-221.

129. Singer E, Valdes-Sueiras M, Commins D, Levine A. Neurologic Presentations of AIDS. *Neurol Clin.* 2010;28(1):253-275.

130. Matinella A, Lanzafame M, Bonometti MA, et al. Neurological complications of HIV infection in pre-HAART and HAART era: a retrospective study. *J Neurol.* 2015;262(5):1317-1327.

131. Reger M, Welsh R, Razani J, Martin D, Boone K. A meta-analysis of the neuropsychological sequelae of HIV infection. *J Int Neuropsychol Soc.* 2002;8(3):410-424.

132. McArthur J. HIV dementia: an evolving disease. *J Neuroimmunol.* 2004;157(1-2):3-10.

133. Brew B. Evidence for a change in AIDS dementia complex in the era of highly active antiretroviral therapy and the possibility of new forms of AIDS dementia complex. *AIDS.* 2004;18(Suppl 1):S75-S78.

134. Garvey L, Winston A, Walsh J, et al. HIV-associated central nervous system diseases in the recent combination antiretroviral therapy era. *Eur J Neurol.* 2011;18(3):527-534.

135. Berger J, Pall L, Lanska D, Whiteman M. Progressive multifocal leukoencephalopathy in patients with HIV infection. *J Neurovirol.* 1998;4(1):59-68.

136. Engsig F, Hansen A, Omland L, et al. Incidence, clinical presentation, and outcome of progressive multifocal leukoencephalopathy in HIV-infected patients during the highly active antiretroviral therapy era: a nationwide cohort study. *J Infect Dis.* 2009;199(1):77-83.

137. Griffiths P. Cytomegalovirus infection of the central nervous system. *Herpes.* 2004;11(Suppl 2):95A-104A.

138. Holbrook JT, Colvin R, van Natta ML, Thorne JE, Bardsley M, Jabs DA. Evaluation of the United States public health service guidelines for discontinuation of anticytomegalovirus therapy after immune recovery in patients with cytomegalovirus retinitis. *Am J Ophthalmol.* 2011;152(4):628-637 e621.

139. Jarvis J, Harrison T. HIV-associated cryptococcal meningitis. *AIDS.* 2007;21(16):2119-2129.

140. Perfect JR, Dismukes WE, Dromer F, et al. Clinical practice guidelines for the management of cryptococcal disease: 2010 update by the Infectious Diseases Society of America. *Clin Infect Dis.* 2010;50(3):291-322.

141. Kiderlen TR, Liesenfeld O, Schurmann D, Schneider T. Toxoplasmic encephalitis in AIDS-patients before and after the introduction of highly active antiretroviral therapy (HAART). *Eur J Clin Microbiol Infect Dis.* 2011;30(12):1521-1525.

142. Ho Y, Sun H, Chen M, Hsieh M, Sheng W, Chang S. Clinical presentation and outcome of toxoplasmic encephalitis in patients with human immunodeficiency virus type 1 infection. *J Microbiol Immunol Infect.* 2008;41(5):386-392.

143. Bayraktar S, Bayraktar UD, Ramos JC, Stefanovic A, Lossos IS. Primary CNS lymphoma in HIV positive and negative patients: comparison of clinical characteristics, outcome and prognostic factors. *J Neurooncol.* 2011;101(2):257-265.

144. Riedel D, Pardo C, McArthur J, Nath A. Therapy Insight: CNS manifestations of HIV-associated immune reconstitution inflammatory syndrome. *Nat Clin Pract Neurol.* 2006;2(10):557-565.

145. Shelburne S, Visnegarwala F, Darcourt J. Incidence and risk factors for immune reconstitution inflammatory syndrome during highly active antiretroviral therapy. *AIDS*. 2005;19(4):399-406.

146. Robertson J, Meier M, Wall J, Ying J, Fichtenbaum C. Immune reconstitution syndrome in HIV: validating a case definition and identifying clinical predictors in persons initiating antiretroviral therapy. *Clin Infect Dis*. 2006;42(11):1639-1646.

147. Johnson T, Nath A. Immune reconstitution inflammatory syndrome and the central nervous system. *Curr Opin Neurol*. 2011;24(3):284-290.

148. de Boer IM, Prins JM, Sprangers MA, Smit C, Nieuwkerk PT. Self-reported symptoms among HIV-Infected patients on highly active antiretroviral therapy in the ATHENA cohort in The Netherlands. *HIV Clin Trials*. 2011;12(3):161-170.

149. Silverberg MJ, Ray GT, Saunders K, et al. Prescription long-term opioid use in HIV-infected patients. *Clin J Pain*. 2012;28(1):39-46.

150. Breitbart W, Passik S, McDonald MV, et al. Patient-related barriers to pain management in ambulatory AIDS patients. *Pain*. 1998;76(1-2):9-16.

151. Singer EJ, Zorilla C, Fahy-Chandon B, Chi S, Syndulko K, Tourtellotte WW. Painful symptoms reported by ambulatory HIV-infected men in a longitudinal study. *Pain*. 1993;54(1):15-19.

152. Cedeno-Laurent F, Gomez-Flores M, Mendez N, et al. New insights into HIV-1-primary skin disorders. *J Int AIDS Soc*. 2011;14:5.

153. Maurer TA. Dermatologic manifestations of HIV infection. *Top HIV Med*. 2005;13(5):149-154.

154. Berman B, Flores F, Burke G, 3rd. Efficacy of pentoxifylline in the treatment of pruritic papular eruption of HIV-infected persons. *J Am Acad Dermatol*. 1998;38(6 Pt 1):955-959.

155. Annam V, Yelikar B, Inamadar A, Palit A, Arathi P. Clinicopathological study of itchy folliculitis in HIV-infected patients. *Indian J Dermatol Venereol Leprol*. 2010;76(3):259-262.

156. Brazzelli V, Barbagallo T, Prestinari F, Ciocca O, Vassallo C, Borroni G. HIV seronegative eosinophilic pustular folliculitis successfully treated with doxycycline. *J Eur Acad Dermatol Venereol*. 2004;18(4):467-470.

157. Rajendran P, High W, Maurer T. HIV-associated eosinophilic folliculitis. *UpToDate*. www.uptodate.com/contents/hiv-associated-eosinophilic-folliculitis. Accessed June 27, 2017.

158. Osei-Sekyere B, Karstaedt AS. Immune reconstitution inflammatory syndrome involving the skin. *Clin Exp Dermatol*. 2010;35(5):477-481.

159. Mangili A, Murman DH, Zampini AM, Wanke CA. Nutrition and HIV infection: review of weight loss and wasting in the era of highly active antiretroviral therapy from the nutrition for healthy living cohort. *Clin Infect Dis*. 2006;42(6):836-842.

160. Kotler DP, Tierney AR, Wang J, Pierson RN, Jr. Magnitude of body-cell-mass depletion and the timing of death from wasting in AIDS. *Am J Clin Nutr*. 1989;50(3):444-447.

161. Shikuma CM, Zackin R, Sattler F, et al. Changes in weight and lean body mass during highly active antiretroviral therapy. *Clin Infect Dis*. 2004;39(8):1223-1230.

162. Davis M, Lasheen W, Walsh D, Mahmoud F, Bicanovsky L, Lagman R. A phase II dose titration study of thalidomide for cancer-associated anorexia. *J Pain Symptom Manage*. 2011.

163. Grinspoon S. Management of tissue wasting in patients with HIV infection. *UpToDate*. www.uptodate.com/contents/management-of-tissue-wasting-in-patients-with-hiv-infection. Accessed August 2, 2011.

164. Falutz J. Growth hormone and HIV infection: contribution to disease manifestations and clinical implications. *Best Pract Res Clin Endocrinol Metab*. 2011;25(3):517-529.

165. Farrar DJ. Megestrol acetate: promises and pitfalls. *AIDS Patient Care STDS*. 1999;13(3):149-152.

166. Stein M, O'Sullivan P, Wachtel T, et al. Causes of death in persons with human immunodeficiency virus infection. *Am J Med*. 1992;93(4):387-390.

167. Kravcik S, Hawley-Foss N, Victor G, et al. Causes of death of HIV-infected persons in Ottawa, Ontario, 1984-1995. *Arch Intern Med.* 1997;157(18):2069-2073.

168. Shiels M, Pfeiffer R, Gail M, et al. Cancer burden in the HIV-infected population in the United States. *J Natl Cancer Inst.* 2011;103(9):753-762.

169. Bower M, Palmieri C, Dhillon T. AIDS-related malignancies: changing epidemiology and the impact of highly active antiretroviral therapy. *Curr Opin Infect Dis.* 2006;19(1):14-19.

170. Cianfrocca M, Lee S, Von Roenn J, et al. Randomized trial of paclitaxel versus pegylated liposomal doxorubicin for advanced human immunodeficiency virus-associated Kaposi sarcoma: evidence of symptom palliation from chemotherapy. *Cancer.* 2010;116(16):3969-3977.

171. Simard EP, Pfeiffer RM, Engels EA. Cumulative incidence of cancer among individuals with acquired immunodeficiency syndrome in the United States. *Cancer.* 2011;117(5):1089-1096.

172. Engels EA, Rosenberg PS, Frisch M, Goedert JJ. Cancers associated with Kaposi's sarcoma (KS) in AIDS: a link between KS herpes virus and immunoblastic lymphoma. *Br J Cancer.* 2001;85(9):1298-1303.

173. Spagnuolo V, Galli L, Salpietro S, et al. Ten-year survival among HIV-1 infected subjects with AIDS- or non-AIDS-defining malignancies. *Int J Cancer.* 2012;130(12):2990-2996.

174. Herida M, Mary-Krause M, Kaphan R, et al. Incidence of non-AIDS-defining cancers before and during the highly active antiretroviral therapy era in a cohort of human immunodeficiency virus-infected patients. *J Clin Oncol.* 2003;21(18):3447-3453.

175. Hessol NA, Katz MH, Liu JY, Buchbinder SP, Rubino CJ, Holmberg SD. Increased incidence of Hodgkin disease in homosexual men with HIV infection. *Ann Intern Med.* 1992;117(4):309-311.

176. Malignant lymphomas in patients with or at risk for AIDS in Italy. Italian Cooperative Group for AIDS-Related Tumors. *J Natl Cancer Inst.* 1988;80(11):855-860.

177. Levine AM. Hodgkin's disease in the setting of human immunodeficiency virus infection. *J Natl Cancer Inst Monogr.* 1998(23):37-42.

178. Serraino D, Boschini A, Carrieri P, et al. Cancer risk among men with, or at risk of, HIV infection in southern Europe. *AIDS.* 2000;14(5):553-559.

179. Tirelli U, Errante D, Dolcetti R, et al. Hodgkin's disease and human immunodeficiency virus infection: clinicopathologic and virologic features of 114 patients from the Italian Cooperative Group on AIDS and Tumors. *J Clin Oncol.* 1995;13(7):1758-1767.

180. Vogel M, Friedrich O, Luchters G, et al. Cancer risk in HIV-infected individuals on HAART is largely attributed to oncogenic infections and state of immunocompetence. *Eur J Med Res.* 2011;16(3):101-107.

181. Levine AM. HIV-associated Hodgkin's disease. Biologic and clinical aspects. *Hematol Oncol Clin North Am.* 1996;10(5):1135-1148.

182. Costello R, Heuberger L, Petit N, Olive D, Gastaut JA. Hodgkin's disease in patients infected with the human immunodeficiency virus. *Rev Med Interne.* 1998;19(8):558-564.

183. Vilchez RA, Finch CJ, Jorgensen JL, Butel JS. The clinical epidemiology of Hodgkin lymphoma in HIV-infected patients in the highly active antiretroviral therapy (HAART) era. *Medicine (Baltimore).* 2003;82(2):77-81.

184. Errante D, Gabarre J, Ridolfo AL, et al. Hodgkin's disease in 35 patients with HIV infection: an experience with epirubicin, bleomycin, vinblastine and prednisone chemotherapy in combination with antiretroviral therapy and primary use of G-CSF. *Ann Oncol.* 1999;10(2):189-195.

185. Levine AM, Li P, Cheung T, et al. Chemotherapy consisting of doxorubicin, bleomycin, vinblastine, and dacarbazine with granulocyte-colony-stimulating factor in HIV-infected patients with newly diagnosed Hodgkin's disease: a prospective, multi-institutional AIDS clinical trials group study (ACTG 149). *J Acquir Immune Defic Syndr.* 2000;24(5):444-450.

186. Bohlius J, Schmidlin K, Boue F, et al. HIV-1-related Hodgkin lymphoma in the era of combination antiretroviral therapy: incidence and evolution of CD4 T-cell lymphocytes. *Blood*. 2011;117(23):6100-6108.

187. Spina M, Gabarre J, Rossi G, et al. Stanford V regimen and concomitant HAART in 59 patients with Hodgkin disease and HIV infection. *Blood*. 2002;100(6):1984-1988.

188. Hartmann P, Rehwald U, Salzberger B, et al. BEACOPP therapeutic regimen for patients with Hodgkin's disease and HIV infection. *Ann Oncol*. 2003;14(10):1562-1569.

189. Xicoy B, Ribera JM, Miralles P, et al. Results of treatment with doxorubicin, bleomycin, vinblastine and dacarbazine and highly active antiretroviral therapy in advanced stage, human immunodeficiency virus-related Hodgkin's lymphoma. *Haematologica*. 2007;92(2):191-198.

190. Palefsky JM, Holly EA, Ralston ML, Da Costa M, Greenblatt RM. Prevalence and risk factors for anal human papillomavirus infection in human immunodeficiency virus (HIV)-positive and high-risk HIV-negative women. *J Infect Dis*. 2001;183(3):383-391.

191. Palefsky JM, Gonzales J, Greenblatt RM, Ahn DK, Hollander H. Anal intraepithelial neoplasia and anal papillomavirus infection among homosexual males with group IV HIV disease. *JAMA*. 1990;263(21):2911-2916.

192. Kreuter A, Brockmeyer NH, Hochdorfer B, et al. Clinical spectrum and virologic characteristics of anal intraepithelial neoplasia in HIV infection. *J Am Acad Dermatol*. 2005;52(4):603-608.

193. Palefsky JM, Holly EA, Efirdc JT, et al. Anal intraepithelial neoplasia in the highly active antiretroviral therapy era among HIV-positive men who have sex with men. *AIDS*. 2005;19(13):1407-1414.

194. Ortoski RA, Kell CS. Anal cancer and screening guidelines for human papillomavirus in men. *J Am Osteopath Assoc*. 2011;111(3 Suppl 2):S35-43.

195. Shiels MS, Pfeiffer RM, Hall HI, et al. Proportions of Kaposi sarcoma, selected non-Hodgkin lymphomas, and cervical cancer in the United States occurring in persons with AIDS, 1980-2007. *JAMA*. 2011;305(14):1450-1459.

196. Heard I. Human papillomavirus, cancer and vaccination. *Curr Opin HIV AIDS*. 2011;6(4):297-302.

197. Kojic EM, Kang M, Cespedes MS, et al. Immunogenicity and safety of the quadrivalent human papillomavirus vaccine in HIV-1-infected women. *Clin Infect Dis*. 2014;59(1):127-135.

198. Maiman M, Tarricone N, Vieira J, Suarez J, Serur E, Boyce JG. Colposcopic evaluation of human immunodeficiency virus-seropositive women. *Obstet Gynecol*. 1991;78(1):84-88.

199. Schafer A, Friedmann W, Mielke M, Schwartlander B, Koch MA. The increased frequency of cervical dysplasia-neoplasia in women infected with the human immunodeficiency virus is related to the degree of immunosuppression. *Am J Obstet Gynecol*. 1991;164(2):593-599.

200. Delmas MC, Larsen C, van Benthem B, et al. Cervical squamous intraepithelial lesions in HIV-infected women: prevalence, incidence and regression. European Study Group on Natural History of HIV Infection in Women. *AIDS*. 2000;14(12):1775-1784.

201. Mwanahamuntu MH, Sahasrabuddhe VV, Stringer JS, Parham GP. Integrating cervical cancer prevention in HIV/AIDS treatment and care programmes. *Bull World Health Organ*. 2008;86(8):D-E.

202. Alfa-Wali M, Tait D, Allen-Mersh T, et al. Colorectal cancer in HIV positive individuals: the immunological effects of treatment. *Eur J Cancer*. 2011;47(16):2403-2407.

203. Huang L, Cattamanchi A, Davis JL, et al. HIV-associated Pneumocystis pneumonia. *Proc Am Thorac Soc*. 2011;8(3):294-300.

204. Nissapatorn V. Toxoplasmosis in HIV/AIDS: a living legacy. *Southeast Asian J Trop Med Public Health*. 2009;40(6):1158-1178.

205. Liu Y. Demonstrations of AIDS-associated malignancies and infections at FDG PET-CT. *Ann Nucl Med*. 2011;25(8):536-546.

206. Lee YC, Wang JT, Sun HY, Chen YC. Comparisons of clinical features and mortality of cryptococcal meningitis between patients with and without human immunodeficiency virus infection. *J Microbiol Immunol Infect*. 2011;44(5):338-345.

207. Boulware DR, Meya DB, Bergemann TL, et al. Clinical features and serum biomarkers in HIV immune reconstitution inflammatory syndrome after cryptococcal meningitis: a prospective cohort study. *PLoS Med*. 2010;7(12):e1000384.

208. Lawn SD, Torok ME, Wood R. Optimum time to start antiretroviral therapy during HIV-associated opportunistic infections. *Curr Opin Infect Dis*. 2011;24(1):34-42.

209. Centers for Disease Control and Prevention, Health Resources and Services Administration, National Institute on Drug Abuse, Substance Abuse and Mental Health Services Administration. *HIV Prevention: Medical Advice for Persons Who Inject Illicit Drugs*. Washington, DC: US Department of Health and Human Services Public Health Service; 1997.

210. Kaplan JE, Benson C, Holmes KH, et al. Guidelines for prevention and treatment of opportunistic infections in HIV-infected adults and adolescents: recommendations from CDC, the National Institutes of Health, and the HIV Medicine Association of the Infectious Diseases Society of America. *MMWR Recomm Rep*. 2009;58(RR-4):1.

211. Hershow RC, Kalish LA, Sha B, Till M, Cohen M. Hepatitis C virus infection in Chicago women with or at risk for HIV infection: evidence for sexual transmission. *Sex Transm Dis*. 1998;25(10):527-532.

212. Alter MJ, Kruszon-Moran D, Nainan OV, et al. The prevalence of hepatitis C virus infection in the United States, 1988 through 1994. *N Engl J Med*. 1999;341(8):556-562.

213. Merwat S, Vierling J. HIV infection and the liver: the importance of HCV-HIV coinfection and drug-induced liver injury. 2011;15(1):131-152.

214. van de Laar TJ, Matthews GV, Prins M, Danta M. Acute hepatitis C in HIV-infected men who have sex with men: an emerging sexually transmitted infection. *AIDS*. 2010;24(12):1799-1812.

215. Greub G, Ledergerber B, Battegay M. Clinical prgression, survival and immune recovery during antiretroviral therapy in patients with HIV-1 and hepatitis C coinfection: the Swiss cohort study. *Lancet*. 2000;356(9244):1800-1805.

216. Poles MA, Dieterich DT. Hepatitis C virus/human immunodeficiency virus coinfection: clinical management issues. *Clin Infect Dis*. 2000;31(1):154-161.

217. Ragni M. Hepatitis C virus/human immunodeficiency virus coinfection: clinical management issues [abstract]. *7th Conf Retrovir Oppor Infect*. 2000;7:129. Abstract 281.

218. Thomas DL, Astemborski J, Rai RM, et al. The natural history of hepatitis C virus infection: host, viral, and environmental factors. *JAMA*. 2000;284(4):450-456.

219. Ockenga J, Tillmann HL, Trautwein C, Stoll M, Manns MP, Schmidt RE. Hepatitis B and C in HIV-infected patients. Prevalence and prognostic value. *J Hepatol*. 1997;27(1):18-24.

220. Leone S, Gregis G, Quinzan G, et al. Causes of death and risk factors among HIV-infected persons in the HAART era: analysis of a large urban cohort. *Infection*. 2011;39(1):13-20.

221. Justice A, Chang C, Becker S, Faffanti S, Fusco J, West N. Sensitivity of CD4 cell count and viral load for predicting mortality in the post-HAART era [abstract]. *Abstr Intersci Conf Antimicrob Agents Chemother*. 1999;39:455. Abstract 125.

222. Shepherd J, Brodin H, Cave C, Waugh N, Price A, Gabbay J. Pegylated interferon alpha-2a and -2b in combination with ribavirin in the treatment of chronic hepatitis C: a systematic review and economic evaluation. *Health Technol Assess*. 2004;8(39):iii-iv, 1-125.

223. Michielsen P, Bottieau E, Van Vlierberghe H, et al. Treatment of chronic hepatitis C in patients with human immunodeficiency virus (HIV) with weekly peginterferon alpha-2b plus ribavirin: a multi-centred Belgian study. *Acta Gastroenterol Belg.* 2009;72(4):389-393.

224. Masia M, Robledano C, Lopez N, Escolano C, Gutierrez F. Treatment for hepatitis C virus with pegylated interferon-alpha plus ribavirin induces anti-atherogenic effects on cardiovascular risk biomarkers in HIV-infected and -uninfected patients. *J Antimicrob Chemother.* 2011;66(8):1861-1868.

225. Lekas HM, Siegel K, Leider J. Challenges Facing Providers Caring for HIV/HCV-Coinfected Patients. *Qual Health Res.* 2011.

226. Osilla KC, Wagner G, Garnett J, et al. Patient and provider characteristics associated with the decision of HIV coinfected patients to start hepatitis C treatment. *AIDS Patient Care STDS.* 2011;25(9):533-538.

227. Singal AK, Anand BS. Management of hepatitis C virus infection in HIV/HCV co-infected patients: clinical review. *World J Gastroenterol.* 2009;15(30):3713-3724.

228. Lugassy DM, Farmer BM, Nelson LS. Metabolic and hepatobiliary side effects of antiretroviral therapy (ART). *Emerg Med Clin North Am.* 2010;28(2):409-419.

229. Berger A, Shuster J, Von Roenn J. *Principles and Practice of Palliative Care and Supportive Oncology.* Philadelphia, PA: Lippincott Williams and Wilkins; 2006.

230. Munoz-Moreno JA, Fumaz CR, Prats A, et al. Interruptions of antiretroviral therapy in human immunodeficiency virus infection: are they detrimental to neurocognitive functioning? *J Neurovirol.* 2010;16(3):208-218.

231. Goforth HW, Lowery J, Cutson TM, McMillan ES, Kenedi C, Cohen MA. Impact of bereavement on progression of AIDS and HIV infection: a review. *Psychosomatics.* 2009;50(5):433-439.

232. Munro I, Edward KL. The burden of care of gay male carers caring for men living with HIV/AIDS. *Am J Mens Health.* 2010;4(4):287-296.

233. Glackin M, Higgins A. The grief experience of same-sex couples within an Irish context: tacit acknowledgement. *Int J Palliat Nurs.* 2008;14(6):297-302.

234. Rando TA. *Treatment of Complicated Mourning.* Champaign, IL: Research Press; 1993.

235. Bristowe K, Marshall S, Harding R. The bereavement experiences of lesbian, gay, bisexual and/or trans* people who have lost a partner: A systematic review, thematic synthesis and modelling of the literature. *Palliat Med.* 2016;30(8):730-744.

236. Nord D. Issues and implications in the counseling of survivors of multiple AIDS-related loss. *Death Stud.* 1996;20(4):389-413.

237. Smith NG, Tarakeshwar N, Hansen NB, Kochman A, Sikkema KJ. Coping mediates outcome following a randomized group intervention for HIV-positive bereaved individuals. *J Clin Psychol.* 2009;65(3):319-335.

238. Hansen NB, Vaughan EL, Cavanaugh CE, Connell CM, Sikkema KJ. Health-related quality of life in bereaved HIV-positive adults: relationships between HIV symptoms, grief, social support, and Axis II indication. *Health Psychol.* 2009;28(2):249-257.

239. Pereira SM, Fonseca AM, Carvalho AS. Burnout in palliative care: a systematic review. *Nurs Ethics.* 2011;18(3):317-326.

240. Swetz KM, Harrington SE, Matsuyama RK, Shanafelt TD, Lyckholm LJ. Strategies for avoiding burnout in hospice and palliative medicine: peer advice for physicians on achieving longevity and fulfillment. *J Palliat Med.* 2009;12(9):773-777.

241. Centers for Disease Control and Prevention, US Department of Health and Human Services. Pre-exposure prophylaxis (PrEP). https://www.cdc.gov/hiv/risk/prep/index.html. Accessed January 3, 2017.

242. US Public Health Service. Preexposure Prophylaxis for the Prevention of HIV Infection in the United States—2014: A Clinical Practice Guideline. Washington, DC: Centers for Disease Control and Prevention, US Department of Health and Human Services; 2014. https://www.cdc.gov/hiv/pdf/prepguidelines2014.pdf. Accessed June 28, 2017.

243. Centers for Disease Control and Prevention, US Department of Health and Human Services. Occupational HIV Transmission and Prevention among Health Care Workers. 2016; https://www.cdc.gov/hiv/workplace/healthcareworkers.html. Accessed June 26, 2017.

244. Panlilio A, Cardo D, Grohskopf L, Heneine W, Ross C. Updated US public health service guidelines for the management of occupational exposures to HIV and recommendations for postexposure prophylaxis. *MMWR Morb Mortal Wkly Rep.* 2005;54(RR09):1-17. www.cdc.gov/mmwr/preview/mmwrhtml/rr5409a1.htm. Accessed June 28, 2017.

# Dementia

*Dementia* is an acquired loss of memory that is substantial enough to interfere with everyday functioning plus impairment of at least one other cognitive domain. Given its prolonged course and associated behavioral and psychological symptoms, the care of people with dementia presents numerous opportunities to integrate palliative care from diagnosis to end of life. Each stage of the disease (mild, moderate, severe, and end stage) reflects a decline in cognitive and functional abilities for which palliative interventions can improve outcomes and quality of life (QOL). With the growing prevalence of dementia, palliative medicine clinicians will care for increasing numbers of patients with dementia either as a primary diagnosis or as a condition that coexists with other life-limiting conditions. In addition to caring for patients, clinicians also need to tend to caregivers' well-being because they play a vital role in the health of people with dementia. Therefore, a palliative model should focus on both the patient and caregiver's physical, psychological, social, and spiritual care. The nature and focus of care is modified over time as a patient's memory loss and functional dependence progress and caregivers' roles change.

## Diagnosis and Meaningful Subtypes

**Table 9** lists some of the more common etiologies of dementia for which an accurate clinical diagnosis relies on strict and validated criteria. During the past decade, characteristic symptoms of the various subtypes of dementia have been found to correspond with pathological changes in the brain (eg, protein deposition, ischemia).[1] These changes in the brain, along with an individual's life experiences and comorbid conditions, influence prognosis, symptomatology, treatment, and expected disease course. As a dementia progresses, clinical symptoms become remarkably similar among the various subtypes, making an etiology-based diagnosis more difficult. In the more advanced stages of dementia, a patient's prognosis, symptoms, and treatment decisions overlap considerably, resulting in a more consistent management approach.

Chronic traumatic encephalopathy (CTE) is emerging as a much discussed but rare disease process that is characterized as a progressive degenerative disease of the brain found in athletes (and others) with a history of repetitive brain trauma, including symptomatic concussions as well as asymptomatic subconcussive hits to the head. A CTE diagnosis can only be determined during autopsy by studying sections of the brain. It is a controversial condition that is not well understood. Researchers do not yet know the frequency of CTE in the population and do not understand the causes.[2] There is no cure.

Memory changes that occur with advanced age can be conceptualized as existing on a continuum: normal changes, mild cognitive impairment (mild neurocognitive disorder per the *Diagnostic and Statistical Manual of Mental Disorders,* 5th ed. [*DSM-5*]), and dementia (major neurocognitive disorder per *DSM-5*). For example, it is normal for older adults to need more

## Table 9. Most Common Etiologies of Dementia in the United States

| Dementia Diagnosis | Relative Frequency | Pathophysiology |
| --- | --- | --- |
| Alzheimer's disease (AD) | 35% | Beta-amyloid plaques and neuro-fibrillary tangles (tau) |
| Mixed (vascular disease and AD) | 15% | Combination of AD and vascular disease |
| Lewy body dementia | 15% | Alpha-synuclein protein |
| Vascular dementia | 10% | Cortical infarcts, subcortical infarcts, and leukoaraiosis (also known as white matter hyperintensities on magnetic resonance imaging) |
| Frontotemporal dementia (Pick's disease) | 5% | Tau protein |

Note: Studies indicate that 55% to 70% of dementia cases have a significant component of AD that often coexists with Lewy body dementia and vascular dementia.

time to learn new information, but older adults can retain the same amount of information as younger people.[3] Patients with mild cognitive impairment (mild neurocognitive disorder) exhibit abnormalities in memory or one other cognitive domain (ie, aphasia, agnosia, apraxia, executive functioning). Other areas of cognition, however, remain intact, and the cognitive deficit does not impair functional abilities. Early recognition, however, allows for appropriate evaluation, diagnosis, and treatment as well as providing education, psychosocial support, and advance care planning. The presence of mild cognitive impairment puts people at high risk for developing dementia within several years' time.[4] The International Association of Gerontology and Geriatrics Global Aging Research Network (IAGG GARN) consensus panel examined the importance of early recognition of impaired cognitive health. Their major conclusion was that case finding by physicians and healthcare professionals is an important step toward enhancing brain health for aging populations throughout the world. This conclusion is consistent with the position of the Centers for Medicare and Medicaid Services (CMS), which reimburses for detection of cognitive impairment as part the of Medicare Annual Wellness Visit, and with the international call for early detection of cognitive impairment as a patient's right. The panel agreed on the following specific findings:

- Validated screening tests are available that take 3 to 7 minutes to administer.
- A combination of patient- and informant-based screens is the most appropriate approach for identifying early cognitive impairment.
- Early cognitive impairment may have treatable components.
- Emerging data support a combination of medical and lifestyle interventions as a potential way to delay or reduce cognitive decline.

Although many types of dementia exist, most patients with dementia have Alzheimer's disease (AD), vascular dementia, Lewy body dementia, or some combination of these conditions.[5]

AD is the most common cause of dementia in the United States, with a molecular pathogenesis of protein deposition—namely, beta-amyloid plaques and neurofibrillary tangles (tau).[6] The hippocampus and neocortex are the primary affected sites that translate into clinical manifestations of the disease. A clinical diagnosis using validated criteria is correct more than 85% of the time at postmortem examination.[7] The *DSM-5* criteria for major cognitive disorder is evidence of significant cognitive decline in memory or another cognitive ability, such as language or learning, that interferes with independence in everyday activities. The cognitive dysfunction must be severe enough to impair social or occupational functioning and cannot be attributed to another cognitive disorder.[8] Mild neurocognitive disorder was introduced in *DSM-5*. Mild neurocognitive disorder is very similar to mild cognitive impairment (MCI); for the clinician, the two entities are equivalent. Mild neurocognitive disorder refers to a condition involving cognitive impairment in one or more domains, often memory, with relative preservation of activities of daily living (ADLs) and the absence of dementia.

One of the first symptoms of AD is memory loss, particularly difficulty encoding new memories. As the disease progresses, patients begin to experience disorganized thoughts, confusion, and disorientation. At the same time, affected people begin to have language difficulties, such as substituting words and forgetting the names of objects. Executive functioning also becomes impaired, which results in impaired judgment. In addition to cognitive decline, noncognitive behavioral and psychological symptoms, including agitation, psychosis, and mood disorders (predominantly depression), frequently develop.[9]

The Alzheimer's Association and National Institutes of Health have proposed modifying AD diagnostic criteria. This modification includes updated criteria for AD, the designation of mild cognitive impairment likely attributable to AD, and new criteria for people with evidence of preclinical disease. The proposed modifications are intended to incorporate significant scientific advances, which include the application of biomarkers obtained from cerebrospinal fluid and the application of newer neuroimaging techniques.[10] The former builds upon evidence that early amyloid deposition in the brain (low cerebrospinal fluid amyloid beta-1-42) leads to neuronal damage (high cerebrospinal fluid tau) and subsequent neurodegeneration (loss of neuronal tissue). Low amyloid and high tau in the cerebrospinal fluid indicate the development or presence of AD. The latter incorporates structural and functional imaging to identify changes within the brain suggestive of the presence or evolution (preclinical stage) of AD.[11] Tracers developed for positron emission tomography (PET) to assess for amyloid deposits *in vivo*, such as Pittsburgh compound B, serve as an example of imaging to detect AD's preclinical stage. Amyloid deposits evident on scan in cognitively intact people have been found to predict a higher risk for developing AD years after the scan.

Vascular dementia is the second most common form of dementia in the United States.[12] The etiology of neuronal loss or dysfunction causing vascular cognitive impairment includes cortical infarcts, subcortical infarcts, and leukoaraiosis (damage to the cerebral white matter appearing as hyperintensities or bright spots on magnetic resonance imaging [MRI]).[13,14] The manifestations of cognitive loss are variable and depend on the location and extent of the underlying lesions. Vascular dementia and AD often coexist; the presence of vascular disease appears to predispose the clinical expression of AD, especially among older adults.[15]

Lewy body dementia, another frequent cause of cognitive dysfunction, occurs as a result of alpha-synuclein protein deposition in the cortex and subcortex. Patients exhibit memory loss and deficits in attention, executive functioning, and visuospatial ability.[16,17] A diagnosis of Lewy body dementia includes the presence of core and suggestive features. The core features of the disease include fluctuating cognition with pronounced variations in attention and alertness, recurrent visual hallucinations that typically are well formed and detailed, and spontaneous features of parkinsonism. Suggestive features of the disease include rapid eye movement (REM) sleep behavior disorder, severe neuroleptic sensitivity, and low-dopamine transporter uptake in the basal ganglia on functional imaging. Supportive features such as repeated falls and syncope, transient and unexplained loss of consciousness, and severe autonomic dysfunction are commonly present but lack diagnostic specificity. The presence of Lewy body dementia and parkinsonian symptoms should occur around the same time to differentiate between people with Lewy body dementia and those with Parkinson's disease (PD) who eventually develop dementia years after diagnosis.

Current recommendations for diagnostic testing include screening for vitamin $B_{12}$ deficiency and thyroid disorders, which, if present, may contribute to additional morbidity. Routine screening for syphilis generally is not recommended unless the patient represents a population with a high prevalence of the disease. Physicians should consider neuroimaging if dementia presents with atypical features or if a clinician determines the need based on a history of falls, a focal neurologic examination, or other factors. Although reversible causes of dementia are rare, consideration of potential contributors to cognitive loss (eg, metabolic disorders, drugs, medications, toxins, hepatic disease, kidney disease, vitamin deficiencies, endocrinopathies), psychiatric disease (especially depression), and infectious diseases (eg, acquired immune deficiency syndrome, syphilis, Lyme disease) may lead to discovery of additional morbidities associated with cognitive loss. Screening for additional contributors is individualized based on the patient's history and physical examination.

## Epidemiology

Age is the greatest risk factor for dementia; its incidence and prevalence increase dramatically in those older than 65 years. Specifically AD affects 2% to 3% of people older than 65 years and doubles in incidence for every 5 years of age thereafter. As a result, AD prevalence approaches 50% among those older than 85 years.[18] In a 2016 study conducted by the Alzheimer's Association, more than 5 million people in the United States were reported to have AD, and a person develops the disease every 66 seconds.[19] Because the population of people older than 65 years is growing, the number of Americans with AD is projected to climb to 13.1 million by 2050.

The rate of deaths attributable to AD continues to rise dramatically. AD is the fifth leading cause of death for people 65 years and older. According to the Centers for Disease Control and Prevention (CDC), AD deaths rose by 46% between 2000 and 2006, whereas deaths from heart disease, cerebrovascular disease, and many malignancies declined during the same period.[19]

People with AD often have coexisting morbidities including hypertension, heart disease, arthritis, diabetes, peripheral vascular disease, and chronic obstructive pulmonary disease.[20] Consequently, in addition to the cognitive symptoms of AD, patients frequently experience symptoms such as shortness of breath, depression, and pain.[21] As dementia progresses, identifying these physical and psychological conditions becomes challenging, and clinicians need to combine evaluations of caregiver reports and direct observation to optimally assess a patient's well-being.

The financial burden of caring for a person with AD falls on caregivers, employers, and society. The 2016 *Alzheimer's Disease Facts and Figures,* published by the Alzheimer's Association, summarizes the economic impact of dementia in the United States.[19] The direct and indirect cost of AD and other dementias amounts to more than $221.3 billion annually and does not include the contributions of unpaid caregivers, which is estimated to be nearly equal. Caregivers of patients with dementia cost employers $6.5 billion annually in lost productivity, missed work, and replacement workers.[19] Healthcare costs are significantly higher for patients with dementia, and this cost rises substantially as the severity of the condition increases.

## Clinical Situation

### Lucja

Lucja is an 80-year-old woman with arthritis who is brought into a physician's office by her 60-year-old son, Pawel, who has concerns about her memory. Lucja is widowed and lives alone in a senior citizen housing development. Lucja's neighbor called Pawel, who resides in a different state, because her phone service had been discontinued as a result of several unpaid bills. Other neighbors had noticed Lucja appearing "lost" in the supermarket parking lot on multiple occasions and needing help finding her car. Upon visiting his mother, Pawel noticed she had posted several reminder notes throughout her apartment and pots with burned food were sitting in her sink.

When asked about these concerns, Lucja became defensive and said, "I don't know what you are all talking about. I am not crazy!" Although she has been very irritable, she does not have any symptoms of depression, delusions, or hallucinations. She does not drink alcohol, smoke, or use illicit drugs. She is not taking medications and has no other chronic medical conditions. Her physical examination was positive for Myerson's frontal release sign but was otherwise nonfocal. She scored 19 out of 30 on the Mini-Mental State Examination. Laboratory results revealed a normal $B_{12}$ and thyrotropin. A brain computed tomography scan showed small-vessel ischemic changes and diffuse atrophy. Pawel is concerned about his mother's diagnosis.

 The physician should review with Pawel the important parts of Lucja's history, physical exam, and results of testing that lead to the diagnosis of dementia.

 It is important for Lucja's family to understand that while there may be a small amount of uncertainty with the diagnosis, further diagnostic testing at this time will not be helpful.

 A thoughtful and honest conversation will allow Pawel to focus on how to best care for Lucja.

 Resources should be dedicated to extensive education for Pawel and the rest of the family and Lucja's community of caregivers. The focus should be about the nature of the disease, likely course, and management of this condition as well as referrals to available resources in the community including advance care planning for legal, medical, and financial matters.

*Case continues on page 68*

## Disease Trajectory and Management

### *Description of Typical Disease Course*

AD is a terminal illness for which average life expectancy is 4 to 8 years after diagnosis.[19,22-29] Age at diagnosis appears to influence median survival; a 2010 study found that when dementia is diagnosed for people in their 60s, they have a 6- to 7-year average life expectancy, which falls to 1.9 years if the diagnosis occurs at age 90 years or older.[30] Most dementias follow a disease course typical of other chronic illnesses, with gradual deterioration punctuated by substantial cognitive and functional decline, usually as the result of an acute illness.[31,32] During recovery from the acute illness, patients with dementia usually establish a new, lower level of cognitive and physical functioning.[33,34] In the advanced stages of the disease, any downturn—commonly a pneumonia, urinary-tract infection, febrile episode, or eating problem—can become a terminal event.[35-37] In fact, patients with advanced dementia admitted to the hospital with pneumonia or hip fracture had a 6-month mortality rate of 50%, a significantly higher rate than that of cognitively intact controls.[38] Similar to AD, many of the more common causes of dementia, including vascular, Lewy body, and frontotemporal dementias, follow a similar disease course.[39] However, rarer causes of dementia such as Creutzfeldt-Jakob disease follow a much more rapid course of decline, with a life expectancy of months to a few years from disease onset.

The cognitive and functional decline of patients with AD usually follows a typical pattern (**Figure 2**).[32,40] Patients with mild dementia experience short-term memory loss along with personality changes and difficulties with some instrumental activities of daily living (IADLs), such as medication management and driving. As dementia progresses to the moderate stage, marked loss of short-term memory occurs along with a decline in long-term memory. At the same time, patients have difficulty with most IADLs (eg, shopping, meal preparation, housework) and begin to develop difficulty completing complex ADLs such as bathing. When dementia is severe, most memory is lost and patients have difficulty with basic ADLs including toileting, dressing, and transferring. At the end stage, patients mutter few intelligible words, become bed bound, and develop progressive dysphagia. At this point, patients have a limited life expectancy, and consideration of hospice services would be appropriate.

## Figure 2. Progressive Loss of Activities of Daily Living

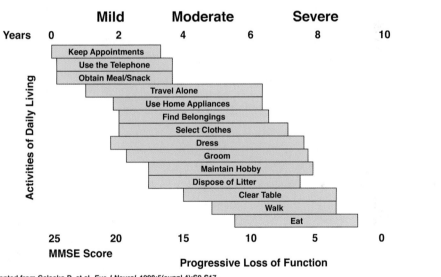

Adapted from Galasko D, et al. *Eur J Neurol.* 1998;5(suppl 4):S9-S17.

*Adapted from An integrated approach to the management of Alzheimer's disease: assessing cognition, function and behavior, by Galasko D, Eur J Neurol, 1998:5(Suppl 4);S9-S17. ©1998 John Wiley and Sons, Inc. Adapted with permission.*

### Treatment Options: Efficacy, Burdens and Benefits, and Potential Rehabilitation
**Pharmacologic**

Given the projected increase in the number of people with AD,[19] efforts have been focused on both prevention and delay of onset. To date, no medical interventions have been found that delay the onset of dementia. Current pharmacologic and nonpharmacologic therapies that ameliorate cognitive and functional decline and decrease challenging behaviors are available but have been shown to be marginally helpful. Good medical care necessitates optimal management of coexisting conditions[20] and ensures that prescribed treatments fit within goals of therapy.[41]

Cholinesterase inhibitors and N-methyl-D-aspartate (NMDA) receptor antagonists are the only two classes of medication approved by the US Food and Drug Administration (FDA) for the treatment of Alzheimer's dementia. Cholinergic neurons innervate areas of the brain involved with memory and learning, and many of the core symptoms of AD can be linked to decreases in cholinergic transmission.[42] Cholinesterase inhibitors are thought to suppress acetylcholinesterase activity, which degrades acetylcholine in the synaptic cleft. As a result, the synaptic levels of acetylcholine increase, improving neurotransmission and attenuating some of AD's cognitive symptoms.

Cholinesterase inhibitors currently available include donepezil, rivastigmine, and galantamine. All three agents are approved by the FDA for the treatment of mild to moderate AD. However, donepezil and rivastigmine are currently approved for the treatment of moderate to severe AD, as well. These agents have slightly different mechanisms of action on acetylcholinesterase, but clinical outcomes are remarkably similar (**Table 10**). FDA approval of these agents requires cognitive benefits and demonstrable differences in global impression of change in favor of the study drug. Donepezil is still the most widely prescribed acetylcholinesterase inhibitor, probably because of its convenient once-a-day dosing, superior tolerability, and approval for all stages of the disease.[43]

For those with mild to moderate Alzheimer's dementia (ie, patients meet standard diagnostic criteria for AD with Mini-Mental State Examination [MMSE] scores of 10 to 26 out of 30, with no other contributing etiology to memory loss), active treatment with cholinesterase inhibitors slows the disease process (cognitive, functional, and behavioral outcomes) compared with placebo.[44-46] Cognitive performance measurement in most of the trials used the Alzheimer's Disease Assessment Scale-Cognitive (ADAS-Cog), a 70-point, 11-item scale that assesses memory, language, orientation, reason, and praxis; a three-point difference over time is considered clinically significant. In general, 15% to 20% of patients in clinical trials showed marked improvement in cognitive performance (ie, a seven-point change in ADAS-Cog scores over time), and 30% displayed some improvement (ie, a three-point change in ADAS-Cog scores over time) compared with placebo over 3 to 6 months. The number needed to treat to obtain the clinical benefit was around 4 to 6, depending on the clinical study. Statistically and clinically significant differences in cognitive performance emerged by 12 weeks and persisted

## Table 10. Medications Commonly Used to Treat Alzheimer's Disease*

| Medication | Mechanism of Action | Disease Severity Indication | Dosage | Side Effects |
|---|---|---|---|---|
| Donepezil (Aricept) | Reversible acetylcholinesterase inhibitor | Mild to moderate; moderate to severe | Mild to moderate: 5 mg-10 mg once daily. Moderate to severe: 10 mg-23 mg once daily. Start 5 mg at bedtime for 4-6 weeks before increasing dose. | Nausea, vomiting, diarrhea (less common), and nightmares; at 23 mg dose, side effects double compared to 10 mg dose |
| Galantamine (Razadyne, Razadyne ER) | Reversible acetylcholinesterase competitive inhibitor (nicotinic modulation, not on current PI) | Mild to moderate | 8 mg-24 mg once daily. Start 4 mg twice daily with meals; may increase every 4 weeks as tolerated or use once daily dosing regimen | Nausea, vomiting, diarrhea, weight loss |
| Rivastigmine (Exelon) | Pseudoirreversible inhibitor of acetylcholinesterase. PI says reversible | Mild, moderate, and severe AD. Mild to moderate dementia associated with PD | 6 mg-12 mg once daily orally; start 1.5 mg twice daily. 4.6 mg once daily by patch; increase to 9.5 mg once daily after 4 weeks; may increase to 13.3 mg/once daily patch after 4 weeks | Nausea and vomiting (more common), diarrhea, weight loss, dizziness. Patch has fewer side effects overall but may be associated with pigment changes on skin. The 4.6 mg/hour dose recommended for persons weighing more than 50kg. |
| Memantine (Namenda) | Noncompetitive antagonist NMDA receptors | Moderate to severe | Target dose is 28 mg once daily; start at 7 mg once daily and increase by 7 mg increments at a minimum of every 7 days to a maximum of 28 mg/day. Only available as a once-daily regimen as Namenda XR | Hypertension, constipation, dizziness, headache. Reduce dose in severe renal impairment; for CrCl 5-29 mL/min, maximum dose is 14 mg/day. |

*CrCl, creatinine clearance; NMDA, n-methyl-d-aspartate; PI, prescribing information*

*\*Namzaric is a once-a-day combination product with 10 mg donepezil and 7/14/21/28 mg of memantine. It may improve compliance; however, it has no other improvements over currently available products and is not available generically.*

until the end of the study (usually 24 weeks). Few of the clinical trials lasted beyond 24 to 36 weeks; however, active treatment continued to be associated with clinically significant benefit compared with placebo in several studies that continued to 1 year.

Studies using donepezil that were designed to specifically assess functional outcomes found that active treatment was associated with a 38% reduction in functional decline, which is defined as an inability to perform one or more ADLs, inability to perform 20% or more of IADLs, or a global worsening in severity of dementia from baseline compared with the placebo group.[47,48] Stated another way, the median time to clinically evident functional decline was 208 days for the placebo group versus 357 days for the donepezil-treated group. The probability of no clinically evident functional decline at 48 weeks was 51% for the donepezil group and 35% for the placebo group.

Neuropsychiatric symptoms also may improve with cholinesterase inhibitor therapy. A meta-analysis of cholinesterase inhibitor trials found that these agents provided a modest benefit that alleviated neuropsychiatric symptoms.[48] The behaviors studied were delusions, hallucinations, agitation, depression, anxiety, euphoria, apathy, disinhibition, irritability, aberrant motor behavior, nighttime behaviors, and appetite and eating disorders. The improvement represents an effect size similar to that of antipsychotic drug trials.[49] A 2007 randomized controlled trial that enrolled subjects with AD and refractory agitation who resided in the nursing home setting found donepezil to be no more effective than placebo in decreasing these behaviors.[50] A 2015 meta-analysis suggests worsening of neuropsychiatric symptoms and cognitions when these agents are discontinued.[51]

Because functional impairment and behavioral disturbances are associated with an increased risk of nursing home placement for people with Alzheimer's dementia and cholinesterase inhibitors improve these patients' cognitive, functional, and behavioral outcomes, it has been hypothesized that use of such agents may delay nursing home placement. One study found that donepezil used at higher dosages (10 mg daily) was associated with a 17.5-month delay in nursing home placement. Another study found that cholinesterase inhibitor therapy significantly reduced the risk of nursing home placement by 28% at 12 months and 21% at 18 months; however, by 36 months the risk of nursing home placement was not statistically different between active therapy and placebo. Taken together, it appears that cholinesterase inhibitor therapy may temporarily delay nursing home placement for people with Alzheimer's dementia.[52,53]

Donepezil and rivastigmine are cholinesterase inhibitors approved for the treatment of moderate to severe AD. Two published double-blind, placebo-controlled, randomized studies found significant benefit with active treatment of donepezil 10 mg daily on cognitive, functional, and global impression of change outcomes.[54,55] A 23-mg formulation has received FDA approval for moderate to severe AD. At this higher dose, participants on average had only a two-point improvement on the Severe Impairment Battery (SIB), which was developed to measure cognition in people with moderate to severe dementia (scores range from 0-100) compared with the 10-mg dose, but participants had about twice the number of side effects, particularly nausea and vomiting, diarrhea, and dizziness.[56]

To date, studies have not included enough hospice-eligible patients to determine whether cholinesterase inhibitors could benefit patients with end-stage dementia. Many experts argue that the likelihood of clinically relevant improvement or disease stabilization in bed-bound, mostly nonverbal patients remains remote. Others argue that patients with end-stage dementia maintain some independent functioning, such as holding up their head without assistance or swallowing food without aspiration, and consequently may benefit from cholinesterase inhibitor therapy.[57] The initiation of these therapies among hospice-eligible patients requires a thoughtful discussion that weighs the goals of care against the likely limited ability of these therapies to stabilize or prevent decline of a person's remaining cognitive and functional abilities. Clinicians often question the impact of discontinuing cholinesterase inhibitors in people with end-stage dementia. Although studies of patients with mild to moderate AD found that discontinuing cholinesterase inhibitor therapy leads to a precipitous cognitive and functional decline to nontreatment levels, investigations have not examined the impact of drug discontinuation in those with advanced dementia. Experts generally recommend tapering cholinesterase inhibitor therapy rather than abrupt discontinuation.

Side effects of cholinesterase inhibitors vary substantially but tend to decrease in frequency over time and occur less in people with advanced dementia. Gastrointestinal side effects including nausea, vomiting, and diarrhea are most common. Nausea occurs in less than 10% of patients who use donepezil but in almost 20% of patients using galantamine and 50% of patients using rivastigmine (oral formulation).[45,46,58,59] Vomiting is infrequent with donepezil and galantamine but occurs in more than 25% of patients who take rivastigmine (oral formulation). Diarrhea may occur with all three agents, although it is reported in fewer than 10% of cases. Weight loss is reported with rivastigmine and galantamine, averaging 2 kg overall. Deprescribing these medications in patients with advanced dementia may improve their appetite and weight. Dizziness is not uncommon but is reported more frequently with rivastigmine. Other less frequent side effects include muscle cramps, abnormal dreams (donepezil), syncope, gastrointestinal bleeding, and urinary incontinence.

Overall, cholinesterase inhibitor therapy has been consistently found to improve cognitive, functional, and behavioral outcomes in people with mild to moderate and moderate to severe AD. Studies in vascular dementia, Lewy body dementia, and PD-related dementia also show some benefit of cholinesterase inhibitor therapy compared with placebo, albeit the effect size tends to be lower.[59-61] For dementia with Lewy body and Parkinson's Disease, cholinesterase inhibitors are effective for cognitive and neuropsychiatric symptoms; rivastigmine has the widest evidence base and is the only one with FDA approval.[62] Despite this proven benefit, some experts believe that cholinesterase inhibitors do not modify the underlying neurodegenerative process, that clinical differences between active therapy and placebo are statistically significant but clinically irrelevant, and that the financial cost (about $400 monthly for brand-name drugs, to as little as $30 monthly for generics as they become more available) and side effects do not justify their ubiquitous use. To support this claim, opponents of cholinesterase inhibitors often cite the AD2000 study, a study conducted in England that was designed to assess the clinical relevance of donepezil therapy. The authors concluded that donepezil was not cost effective and that its benefits were below minimally relevant thresholds.[63] Unfortunately, the applicability of AD2000 study findings are limited because of the study's low participant enrollment; that is, the power calculation estimated that 3,000 participants would need to be enrolled to test the hypothesis that active drug therapy decreases primary outcomes of institutionalization, progress of disability, or the related cost-effectiveness measure. Only 566 (19% of target) participants were recruited into the trial; 76% of them were from a select region of the country.

Glutamate is an excitatory amino acid found in the brain, and with pathological conditions such as AD, there is excessive stimulation of NMDA receptors by glutamate.[64] This overactivation is thought to play a role in AD-related cognitive impairments. Blockage of the NMDA receptor by memantine is thought to modulate, in a voltage-dependent manner, the passage of calcium through the ion channels associated with these receptors. It is believed that memantine prevents the neurotoxicity associated with NMDA receptor overactivation while allowing normal glutamine transmission in the brain.[65]

Two pivotal trials led the FDA to approve memantine for the treatment of moderate to severe AD (MMSE scores of 3-14).[66,67] These trials established the efficacy and safety of memantine monotherapy and combination therapy for patients already taking donepezil. Patients who received active treatment experienced improvement in cognition, functioning, behavior, and global impression of change. Memantine therapy was associated with significantly less deterioration than placebo on the SIB; the mean difference between groups was six points ($P < .001$). However, no difference in response was exhibited between memantine therapy and placebo on the neuropsychiatric inventory. Frequency of adverse events was similar in the active treatment and placebo groups, and there was no difference between memantine and placebo in the frequency of side effects.

The addition of memantine administration for patients with moderate to severe AD who were already taking donepezil resulted in additional patient and caregiver benefits compared with patients continuing on donepezil monotherapy. Statistically significant benefits of active treatment compared with placebo emerged by 4 weeks and persisted over the duration of the study to 24 weeks for both primary outcome measures. As in the previous study, rates of occurrence of adverse events in active treatment and placebo were similar between the two groups, and no difference in frequency of side effects existed between memantine and placebo. In addition, caregivers spent 45.8 fewer hours per month on average caring for patients in the memantine-treated group compared with the placebo group. Moreover, the dropout rate for both studies was higher in the placebo group than in the active treatment arm. Subsequently, donepezil and memantine for moderate-to-severe AD was studied to evaluate whether there was a treatment benefit after the progression to this stage.[68] The conclusion was that in patients with moderate or severe AD, continued treatment with donepezil was associated with cognitive benefits that exceeded the minimum clinically important difference and with significant functional benefits over the course of 12 months. However, there were no significant benefits of the combination of donepezil and memantine over donepezil alone.

Memantine also has been studied in people with mild to moderate Lewy body dementia (MMSE scores of 10-24) and PD dementia.[69] Compared with placebo, the active treatment group of memantine, 20 mg daily, showed statistically significant improvements in clinical global impression of change and neuropsychiatric behaviors in people with Lewy body dementia but not PD dementia. However, in most of the cognitive testing and functional outcomes, no significant differences emerged between active treatment and placebo with either dementia group. The benefits observed with memantine were mild, with unclear clinical significance. Whether memantine is effective in more advanced stages of Lewy body dementia and PD dementia remains unknown. There are ongoing dietary supplementation studies but currently no successful recommendations.

### Nonpharmacologic

An array of studies testing the benefits of nonpharmacologic therapies on cognitive, functional, and behavioral outcomes for people with dementia continue to be published. Studies to date generally focus on cognitive training, social engagement, and physical health and functioning. In addition to using these measures, healthcare providers should be aware of community resources and support services so they can refer people with dementia and their caregivers to available resources.

Cognitive training appears to be more useful for people with dementia when interventions target global cognitive status rather than specific cognitive domains.[70] Moreover, benefits have been found to increase when cognitive stimulation is combined with cholinesterase inhibitor therapy. One study that targeted specific cognitive domains found some improvements in functioning on select tasks, such as recall of personal information or face-name recall with a cognitive intervention, but the minor improvements noted did not generalize to neuropsychological measures (ie, verbal memory, visual memory, motor speed).[71] Although no approach can prevent cognitive deterioration over a prolonged period of time (eg, 2 years), no treatment is associated with greater and faster deterioration than any other treatment. Another approach being examined reviews patients' neuropsychological profiles and tailors interventions to emphasize an individual's strengths and mediate their weaknesses.

Investigations examining the role of social engagement found that disengagement was associated with an increased risk of cognitive decline.[72] During a 12-year period, older adults with the highest levels of social engagement were 30% less likely to experience a decline in dementia from none to mild, from mild to moderate, or from moderate to severe. Finally, intervention trials designed to foster social and intellectual engagement have helped enhance cognition in subjects with dementia over a short period, but whether these interventions lead to sustainable improvement in cognition and decreased the risk of institutionalization remains to be elucidated.[73]

Neurodegenerative diseases result in impaired mobility and functional decline. Multiple studies have found that exercise is associated with improved flexibility, balance, and strength among community-dwelling older adults and frail nursing home residents. One study conducted a 12-session, combined home exercise and behavioral management intervention involving patients with AD and their caregivers. At 3 months it was found that intervention-group patients exercised more often and had fewer days of restricted activity than control-group patients.[74] At 2 years intervention-group patients continued to have significantly better physical functioning scores. The intervention group also experienced the additional benefit of significantly lower depression scores than the control arm throughout the 2 years of the study. The study's authors concluded the intervention resulted in improved physical and emotional health of the patients with AD. A 2011 systematic review of the effects of physical activity on physical functioning, QOL, and depression found that physical activity interventions improve physical functioning in those with dementia.[75] However, evidence remains unclear as to whether these interventions decrease depression and improve QOL.

## Clinical Situation

### Lucja's Case Continues (Continued from page 60)

Lucja is diagnosed with moderate-stage dementia, most likely of the Alzheimer's type. Her physician starts her on cholinesterase inhibitor therapy, donepezil, 5 mg daily, to minimize side effects, with a plan to increase to the therapeutic dose of 10 mg daily after 4 weeks. Pawel has taken a leave of absence from work to live with his mother while he decides how to best care for her. He now is managing her finances, cooking for her, driving her, and supervising her medication. On follow-up visits it is observed that her irritability has improved on the new medication. Although her symptoms may have improved, it is now important to review with Pawel issues related to caregiving. Social workers and support groups may help him understand how the illness might progress and the steps he needs to take to prepare for her increasing care needs. Discussions about safe and supportive living environments as well as advance care planning need to occur for the well-being of both of them and the rest of the family. Pawel wonders if there are any other medications or therapies available that can be used or will slow down the disease progression.

 Donepezil and rivastigmine are both approved for moderate and severe disease but are not as successful as families would like.

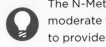

The N-Methyl-D-asparate (NMDA) receptor antagonist memantine (indicated for moderate to severe disease), along with cholinesterase inhibitors, has been shown to provide cognitive, functional, and behavioral benefits compared with placebo in people with moderate AD. As stated previously, studies suggest no significant benefits of the combination of donepezil and memantine over donepezil alone.

Lucja is not showing signs of depression or psychosis, so other medications would not be warranted.

The most important issue to discuss is the inevitability that Lucja will require 24-hour care; therefore, care issues and supportive options should continue to be discussed.

*Case continues on page 83*

## Life Expectancy After Diagnosis

### *Prognostication*

Prognosis in dementia, both at the time of diagnosis and after a person reaches the advanced stage, is an area of much debate and research. Initial studies examining life expectancy for people with dementia suggested median survival is approximately 10 years.[76] However, these studies were limited by including patients into the study at the time of entry instead of at the time of diagnosis, a circumstance that introduced a selection bias. Studies conducted between 1990 and 2010 that ascertain survival at time of diagnosis suggest a much shorter life expectancy, with a mean survival of 4 to 7 years.[22,23,30] Variables associated with shorter survival in these studies included older age at onset, male gender, gait disturbance, wandering, comorbid medical conditions (particularly diabetes, cerebrovascular disease, and cardiovascular disease), a history of falls, and extrapyramidal signs. Survival was not associated with ethnicity, education, behavioral disturbances, dementia diagnosis, or symptoms of depression.

Determining life expectancy is particularly challenging near the end of life and can limit patients' access to hospice enrollment.[77,78] Hospice guidelines currently in use for dementia do a poor job of predicting 6-month mortality and exhibit the greatest variability in survival among all hospice diagnoses (**Table 11**).[79-81] In an effort to improve prediction of 6-month mortality, two risk score models have been developed using nursing home data from the Minimum Data Set: the Mortality Risk Index and Advanced Dementia Prognostic Tool (ADEPT). The Mortality Risk Index retrospectively examined potential variables for which 12 characteristics were identified as predictive of 6-month survival using a derivation and validation cohort (**Table 12**).[82] The authors also compared the effectiveness of their tool with the functional component of the hospice guidelines. The risk score demonstrated better discrimination to

## Table 11. Indicators of Hospice Eligibility for Patients with Dementia Due to Alzheimer's Disease and Related Disorders[84]

Patients are considered to be in the terminal stage of dementia (life expectancy of 6 months or less) if they show all of the following characteristics:
- stage 7 or beyond according to the Functional Assessment Staging Scale (FAST)
- unable to ambulate without assistance
- unable to dress without assistance
- unable to bathe without assistance
- urinary and fecal incontinence, intermittent or constant
- no consistently meaningful verbal communication: stereotypical phrases only or the ability to speak is limited to six or fewer intelligible words.

Patients should have had one of the following within the past 12 months:
- aspiration pneumonia
- pyelonephritis
- septicemia
- decubitus ulcers, multiple, stage 3 or 4
- fever, recurrent after antibiotics
- inability to maintain sufficient fluid and calorie intake with 10% weight loss during the previous 6 months or serum albumin less than 2.5 gm/dL.

*Note: Indicators are specific to Alzheimer's disease and related disorders and are not appropriate for other dementia types. See local coverage determinations (LCDs) for specifics.[85] LCDs vary by Medicare Administrative Contractor (MAC). Use the specific LCD provided by your region's MAC when documenting hospice eligibility.*

## Table 12. Characteristics Associated with 6-Month Mortality Among Nursing Home Residents with Advanced Dementia

| Characteristic | Mortality Risk Multiplier* |
|---|---|
| Complete functional dependence | 1.9 |
| Male gender | 1.9 |
| Cancer diagnosis | 1.7 |
| Oxygen requirement | 1.6 |
| Congestive heart failure | 1.6 |
| Shortness of breath | 1.5 |
| Less than 25% of food consumed | 1.5 |
| Unstable medical condition | 1.5 |
| Bowel incontinence | 1.5 |
| Bed bound | 1.5 |
| Older than 83 years | 1.4 |
| Not awake most of the morning and afternoon | 1.4 |

*Based on the hazard ratio using a stepwise multivariate Cox proportional hazards model.*

predict 6-month mortality; however, the risk tool was not compared with the actual hospice guidelines, which require specific functional limitations and the presence of disease complications (eg, aspiration pneumonia, upper urinary-tract infection, septicemia, multiple decubitus ulcers [stage 3 or 4], recurrent fever despite antibiotics, or inability to take in fluids or food to sustain life).[83] Other limitations of the Mortality Risk Index include the reliance on retrospective data, the participation of only two states, and the inclusion of only recent nursing home admissions.

The ADEPT tool was an attempt to overcome the limitations of the Mortality Risk Index by prospectively collecting information from the Minimum Data Set to develop and validate a prognostic measure while simultaneously gathering clinical information related to hospice eligibility guidelines.[86] The following variables were most predictive of 6-month mortality: nursing home stay less than 90 days, increasing age, male gender, shortness of breath, one or more pressure sores at stage 2 or above, complete functional dependence, bed bound most of day, insufficient oral intake, bowel incontinence, body mass index lower than 18.5, recent weight loss, and congestive heart failure. Risk points were ascribed for each condition based upon the strength of association with 6-month mortality. Risk score ranges were generated and mortality rates within each range calculated. The ADEPT model only performed slightly better than traditional hospice guidelines, with an area under the receiver operating characteristic curve of 0.58 versus 0.55, respectively. As with the Mortality Rate Index, ADEPT was based on nursing home patients and did not incorporate the degree of caregiver support or willingness to pursue interventions such as hospitalization, administration of antibiotics or intravenous fluids, dialysis, or enteral nutrition, which may impact survival.[87]

Overall, efforts to more accurately predict survival among patients with dementia near the end of life have not improved significantly or resulted in newer models, reinforcing the importance of focusing efforts on better delineation of goals of care that reflect a patient's clinical status and previously expressed wishes. It is hoped that hospice, as the current reimbursement structure for state-of-the-art end-of-life care, will consider adopting this focused approach for enrollment because it is more reflective of clinical practice.

### Communication and Hope

Dementia is a progressive illness that gradually robs a person of the ability to communicate. For patients with advanced dementia, nonverbal communication may continue to provide useful information about their symptoms, unmet needs, and experiences up to the time of death. Healthcare providers are called to continue to identify individuals with progressive dementia as a whole person with a spiritual, emotional, social, and physical presence. Through ongoing connection with the family and patient, healthcare providers can continue to offer hope and meaning to their respective experiences and roles.

## Symptom Control

*Pain*

Evaluating the pain experience of a person with dementia can be challenging because of the person's short-term memory impairment and decrements in language and executive functioning. Although cortical processing of pain impulses may be altered, pain pathways in the peripheral and central nervous systems usually are spared from underlying neurodegenerative changes. That is, parenchymal brain changes that lead to cognitive impairment may modify the perception of pain by altering signal processing within the amygdala, thereby decreasing the affective contribution of pain, which in turn lessens reported pain intensity. Despite this theoretical concern, laboratory studies demonstrate that those with mild to moderate cognitive impairment maintain pain thresholds similar to those of cognitively intact populations.[88]

Given that dementia is predominantly a disease affecting older adults, and a large percentage of older adults have chronic medical conditions associated with acute or persistent pain, it is not surprising that pain is such a pervasive symptom among persons with dementia. Cross-sectional studies report a prevalence of pain between 50% and 85% in ambulatory and long-term care settings, respectively.[89-93] Moreover, compared with cognitively intact control groups, patients with cognitive impairment are at higher risk for receiving inadequate analgesia.[94] Many clinicians find it difficult to use several of the drugs available for patients' pain and other symptoms due to safety concerns and report cards for "high-risk" drug use. Arthritis is the second most common chronic condition in all older adults (after hypertension), with 50% of people older than 65 years reporting an arthritis diagnosis and 46% citing chronic joint symptoms.[95] Compounding the problem is that multiple rather than single joint involvement is typical in the older adult population. A 2006 study found that, on average, subjects reported four joints causing pain or stiffness most of the time during the previous 3 months.[96] In addition, many conditions associated with acute pain in older adults, such as postherpetic neuralgia and fractures, lead to persistent pain. See **Table 13** for common conditions associated with noncancer pain in older adults.

A thorough pain assessment for patients with dementia includes patient self-report, caregiver report, consideration of potentially painful morbidities, and direct observation of pain behaviors.[89,97] Pain is a subjective experience that has no objective test, and self-report is the benchmark.[89] Research continues to corroborate data that pain self-report scales demonstrate concurrent validity and reliability in cognitively intact and mildly to moderately impaired patient populations.[90] When asking patients about pain, clinicians should direct questions to the present pain they experience at rest and with activity. As dementia progresses to a more advanced stage, clinicians should continue to ask verbal patients about their present pain experience. At the same time, to ascertain whether a nonverbal patient is experiencing pain, healthcare providers need to incorporate the caregiver's report into their assessment as well as any nonverbal pain indicators from the patient.

## Table 13. Common Conditions Associated with Noncancer Pain in Older Adults

| Condition | Increases in Prevalence with Age |
| --- | --- |
| Osteoarthritis | Yes |
| Crystal arthropathy (gout and pseudogout) | Yes |
| Osteoporosis | Yes |
| Claudication | Yes |
| Postherpetic neuralgia | Yes |
| Spinal stenosis | Yes |
| Fibromyalgia | Yes |
| Diabetic peripheral neuropathy | Probably |
| Constipation | Yes |
| Fractures | Yes |

Observing patients at rest and during activity provides another method to ascertain the pain experience. As dementia progresses to an advanced stage and patients experience substantial memory impairment and language deficits, nonverbal pain indicators become an important assessment tool.[98] To find some of the most commonly used measures with information on validity and reliability, visit http://prc.coh.org/PAIN-NOA.htm (Accessed June 28, 2017). There is consensus among experts supporting the use of the Pain Assessment in Advanced Dementia (PAINAD) and Pain Assessment Checklist for Seniors with Limited Ability to Communicate (PACSLAC) to assess pain in nonverbal nursing home residents.[99] In fact, the group recommended each scale be used to screen for pain behaviors along with direct observation for other common pain behaviors. The PAINAD includes measures of breathing, negative vocalizations, facial expressions, body language, and ability to be consoled. The PACSLAC is organized into behaviors that fall into four groups: facial expressions, activity/body movement, social/personality/mood indicators, and physiologic indicators/sleeping changes/eating/vocal behaviors. Other tools, such as the Checklist of Nonverbal Pain Indicators (CNPI), have not been as extensively validated in assessing persistent pain but maintain good face validity and are easy to use in clinical practice.[100] The CNPI behaviors include nonverbal vocalizations (ie, sighs, gasps, moans, groans, cries), facial grimacing and wincing (ie, furrowed brow, clenched teeth, tightening lips), bracing (ie, holding onto affected area at rest or during movement), rubbing, restlessness (ie, shifting position or inability to keep still), and vocal complaints. Some behaviors included in these scales lack specificity and may be the result of other symptoms or part of the underlying neurodegenerative process.[101] As a result, experts in pain and dementia suggest that if pain is on the differential diagnosis for the observed behavior, an empirical analgesic trial may be indicated.[89,97] With such an approach, an analgesic is prescribed for a specific behavior. Pain is considered a contributor to the behavior if its frequency or severity lessens or if it subsides altogether with analgesia.[102]

Another consideration in pain management is a patient's pain signature.[97] Because pain is a unique and multidimensional experience for each person, patients frequently develop a particular individualized response whenever they experience pain. For instance, a patient in pain may stop eating, refrain from social activities, become agitated, wander, or develop insomnia. In such cases, an analgesic trial may be appropriate to determine whether the patient's change in condition is the result of untreated or undertreated pain. Agitation and pain always need to be separated from delirium. Delirium always has a medical cause, often is multifactorial, rarely is specific, potentially is life-threatening, and can be subtle.

Caregivers can provide a more extensive history of a patient's pain experience, especially as short-term memory worsens. As described in the cancer literature, caregivers of those with mild to moderate dementia report patients having more pain than indicated in self-reports. Caregivers rarely overlook significant pain in patients.[91] At the same time, caregivers can provide valuable information about whether patients are taking prescribed analgesics, and they can describe any side effects.

Professional organizations and experts in the field recommend following the World Health Organization guidelines for cancer pain for the treatment of noncancer pain.[89] Although some controversy exists concerning the use of opioids for noncancer pain in healthier people, those with advanced illness who experience pain should not be denied safe and effective therapy. Opioids can safely and effectively be used to treat suspected pain, even for people with advanced dementia.[103] Many clinicians hesitate to use opioids for patients with dementia for fear their confusion may worsen or they may develop delirium. However, a review article on the cognitive effects of opioids suggests these fears are exaggerated.[104] In fact, evidence suggests opioid use may decrease delirium in some populations.[105] See *UNIPAC 3* for more information on pain management.

## Behavioral and Psychological Symptoms in Dementia
Even though behavioral and psychological symptoms in dementia (BPSD) currently are not included in the diagnostic criteria for AD, noncognitive symptoms represent an important and frequently overlooked aspect of AD care. BPSDs include apathy, affective syndrome (anxiety, depression), psychomotor (agitation, irritability, aberrant motor) behavior, psychosis (delusions and hallucinations), and mania (disinhibition and euphoria); all except affective syndrome show an increase in severity with disease progression.[106,107] In addition to their impact on patients, BPSDs are associated with depression and greater burden for caregivers as well as a higher incidence of institutionalization of those with dementia.[108]

### Mood Disorders
Depression frequently occurs in people with dementia. For mild to moderate dementia, several standardized instruments—including the 30-item Geriatric Depression Scale, the Brief

Carroll Depression Rating Scale, and the Cornell Depression Rating Scale—have been validated.[109-111] For people with moderate to severe dementia, self-report measures are less reliable and valid. Clinicians should consider evaluating for depression if patients experience changes in mood, behavior, cognition, functioning, sleep, or appetite; weight loss; social withdrawal; or apathy. Given the wide variability in the expression of depression in people with advanced dementia and the limited ability of these patients to verbally communicate their experience, an empiric trial of an antidepressant for several weeks may be indicated.[112]

Few studies exist that describe the natural history of depression in dementia. One study that followed patients with mild to moderate dementia monthly for 1 year revealed an annual incidence of 10.6% for major depression and 29.8% for minor depression. Persistent depression lasting 6 months or longer occurred in 20% of patients.[113] Prevalence rates vary widely depending on study population and referral patterns, with major depression affecting 20% to 25% of people with dementia and an additional 20% to 30% of those with minor symptoms.[114,115] In addition to being common, the assessment and management of depression is important because depression negatively influences self-perceived QOL.[116]

Both nonpharmacologic and pharmacologic therapies are appropriate treatment options for depression in those with dementia, but to date few studies have been conducted in either area.[117]

Pharmacologic therapy usually is based on the neuropathological changes associated with depression in patients with Alzheimer's dementia, particularly loss of noradrenergic cells in the locus ceruleus and serotonergic raphe nuclei.[118] Selective serotonin reuptake inhibitors (SSRIs) are considered first-line therapy by some experts because their use has the most data supporting efficacy; however, dosages may need to be increased to obtain optimal effect.[119,120] The tricyclic antidepressant nortriptyline also resulted in clinically significant improvement compared with placebo, but, because of side effects, 34% of participants randomized to active drug therapy had the drug discontinued.[121] Newer agents that maintain dual inhibition of the norepinephrine and serotonin systems have not been studied. One study found the stimulant methylphenidate improved depressive symptoms in dementia. However, clinicians must monitor for psychosis, which can frequently begin or worsen when methylphenidate therapy is initiated in people with dementia.[122,123] Nonpharmacologic therapies that have been successful in decreasing depressive symptoms include cognitive, music, and recreational therapies.[124] Research has not examined the theoretical benefit of combining nonpharmacologic and pharmacologic therapies. A small study has suggested significant clinical benefits with the use of electroconvulsive therapy to manage refractory depression, although people with dementia were significantly more likely to have cognitive decline after 6 months of treatment compared with those without dementia.[125] See *UNIPAC 2* for a general approach to the treatment of depression in those with dementia.

**Apathy**

Apathy frequently is confused with depression. It is a common symptom of AD and other neurodegenerative conditions, with a prevalence higher than 50%.[126] Moreover, it occurs early in the disease course, can persist, and causes significant caregiver distress. Apathy can be defined as a loss of motivation and manifests as diminished initiation, lowered interest, decreasing social engagement, blunted emotions, and lack of insight.[127] Apathy differs from depression in that no symptoms of altered mood are present. Differentiation is important. One study that reviewed the evidence on pharmacological treatments found that the benefits previously reported with acetylcholinesterase inhibitors and memantine were not replicated, and antidepressants have a minimal effect in the treatment of apathy. The use of psychostimulants was inconclusive.[123,127-129]

**Psychosis**

Psychotic symptoms in dementia consist of delusions and hallucinations. Studies conducted between 2002 and 2006 of psychotic symptoms for patients with dementia suggest a point prevalence of delusions between 18% and 35%, whereas hallucinations are reported by 10% to 20% of patients.[130-132] Visual hallucinations are part of the core diagnostic criteria for Lewy body dementia and occur in as many as 77% of patients.[133] Risk factors for developing psychosis include severity of dementia, African American ethnicity, extrapyramidal symptoms, and sensory impairment.[134,135]

Numerous randomized controlled trials and a meta-analysis suggest modest efficacy of antipsychotics over placebo in the treatment of delusions and hallucinations and no apparent efficacy advantage between typical and atypical antipsychotics.[136-138] A 2017 study suggests that placebo is better than antipsychotics.[139] Obviously, treatment tailored to individual patients is paramount. Antipsychotic selection is based on practical considerations such as route of administration and side effect profile. For example, quetiapine is frequently the drug of choice for patients with parkinsonian symptoms, olanzapine and risperidone as a dissolvable wafer can be placed on the tongue for patients who cannot swallow pills, and risperidone liquid can be administered through feeding tubes. **Table 14** lists frequently used atypical antipsychotics and recommended dosages. However, side effects are a notable downside and are perceived to be more numerous with typical antipsychotics. A large randomized controlled trial found increased costs with no improvement in QOL and functional outcomes associated with second-generation antipsychotics for patients with AD and psychosis.[140]

Treatment for delusions and hallucinations with antipsychotics must be carefully considered. This is particularly true for patients with Lewy body dementia, for whom antipsychotics have been associated with marked worsening of rigidity, locked-in syndrome, and even death. For patients with Lewy body dementia and their caregivers, for whom psychosis is particularly bothersome, a trial of the antipsychotic quetiapine (which is considered to cause fewer of these side effects than other antipsychotics) or any of the cholinesterase inhibitors may be indicated. Patients and their caregivers should be assured that these symptoms frequently occur in

# Table 14. Antipsychotic Medications Used for Dementia*

| Antipsychotic | Recommended Dosage | Available Formulations | Frequency | Remarkable Characteristics |
|---|---|---|---|---|
| Haldol | 0.5mg-10 mg per day | Tablet Liquid Intramuscular Subcutaneous Intravenous injections | Twice daily | Extrapyramidal symptoms; dose dependent |
| Risperidone | 0.25 mg-2.0 mg per day | Tablet Disintegrating tablet Liquid Intramuscular injection | Twice daily | Extrapyramidal symptoms; dose dependent |
| Olanzapine | 2.5 mg-15 mg per day | Tablet Disintegrating tablet | Once or twice daily | Weight gain and hyperglycemia more common |
| Quetiapine | 25 mg-400 mg per day | Immediate- or extended-release tablet | Two or three times daily | Fewer extrapyramidal effects; most sedating |
| Aripiprazole | 5 mg-30 mg per day | Tablet Disintegrating tablet Liquid | Once or twice daily | Less likely to prolong QT interval |

*Atypical antipsychotics listed in this table are associated with QT prolongation, weight gain, hyperglycemia, stroke, and death. Newer atypical antipsychotics are not recommended because of the lack of randomized controlled trials in elderly people with dementia. The US Food and Drug Administration (FDA) added black box warnings to several medications commonly used by hospice and palliative care practitioners. Black box warnings are designed to highlight the potential for rare but serious medical complications such as stroke or myocardial infarction associated with the use of these drugs. Hospice and palliative care practitioners should be aware of these FDA black box warnings and the risk-benefit ratio of these medications and alternatives for individual patients. The short prognosis and critical importance of symptom relief for many hospice and palliative care patients may justify the use of these medications despite such risks.*

neurodegenerative diseases, and, if the symptoms are not bothersome to them, pharmacologic therapy likely poses greater risk than close clinical follow-up.[141] Class-related side effects of atypical antipsychotics include weight gain (most concerning with olanzapine), metabolic abnormalities (eg, dyslipidemia, glucose intolerance), QT prolongation, and cerebrovascular events. In a pooled analysis of 3,353 patients on atypical antipsychotics and 1,757 on placebo, active treatment was associated with an increased risk of death (3.5% vs 2.3%, respectively; odds ratio, 1.54 [1.06-2.23]; $P = .02$; risk difference 0.01 [.004-.02]; $P = .01$).[142] Stated another way, for every 100 people treated with an antipsychotic, 9 to 25 will be helped, one or two would suffer cerebrovascular events, and one would die. The FDA added black box warnings to several medications commonly used by hospice and palliative care practitioners. Black box warnings are designed to highlight the potential for rare but serious medical complications such as stroke or myocardial infarction associated with the use of these drugs. Hospice and palliative care practitioners should be aware of these FDA black box warnings and the risk-benefit ratio of these medications and alternatives for individual patients. The short prognosis and critical importance of symptom relief for many hospice and palliative care patients may justify the use of these medications despite such risks. Additional common side effects of typical and atypical antipsychotics include sedation, extrapyramidal effects, edema, and infections.

General principles should be considered before initiating pharmacologic management of psychosis and agitation with antipsychotics. The first step is to try and identify potential contributors to the symptom (eg, anticholinergic medication leading to hallucinations). Next, a thoughtful discussion regarding overall risks and benefits and other treatment options should take place. Identify the target symptom and evaluate other therapies' effectiveness at a specified time point (generally 2-4 weeks). It also is important to use the lowest dosage of medication possible to achieve clinical effectiveness; the prevailing wisdom is to "start low and go slow." Monitor effectiveness and, if the target symptom abates, strongly consider decreasing the medication dose or stopping it altogether. Finally, as with any medication, monitor safety by frequently assessing for side effects. As with any symptomatic therapy, treatment needs to be considered in the context of how bothersome the symptoms are for the patient or caregiver, the goals of care, and the potential benefits compared to risks of the therapy. Consultation with a geriatric psychiatrist may be warranted. The CMS National Partnership to Improve Dementia Care in Nursing Homes focused on reducing the use of antipsychotic medication but also on nonpharmacologic approaches and person-centered care. Nonpharmacologic therapy is less likely to help those with more advanced dementia.[143] CMS also is looking at any adverse consequences of withdrawal of antipsychotics. A study published in 2012 suggests that patients successfully treated with risperidone for 4 to 8 months relapsed after the discontinuation of the drug.[144] Use of antipsychotics in long-term-care facilities for hospice patients is therefore being monitored regardless of the appropriateness of use. Documentation should include (a) that continued use is in accordance with relevant current standards of practice and (b) the clinical rationale for why any attempted dose reduction would be likely to impair the resident's function or cause further psychiatric instability by exacerbating an underlying psychiatric disorder related to life-limiting illness.

## Agitation

Many definitions of the term *agitation* exist and each has relative strengths and weaknesses. Recent studies have indicated the prevalence of agitation throughout a 1-month period among patients with dementia is between 36% and 52%.[130-132] One difficulty with this term is that it is imprecise and can be applied to a variety of conditions such as delirium, depression, terminal symptoms, or a manifestation of the underlying dementia itself. The term does not help distinguish among potential contributing causes that have been established in the literature, including physical symptoms (pain, sleep disturbances), psychological symptoms (depression), medical illness (delirium, seizure disorder, constipation, urinary retention), unmet needs (hunger, social isolation, soiled diaper), environment (unfamiliar surroundings causing fear, overstimulation, or understimulation), medications (theophylline, caffeine, digoxin), and the underlying neurodegenerative process itself (**Table 15**).[145] Also, agitation must be differentiated from resistance to care, which requires a different management approach. To help identify the potential contributors to agitation, healthcare providers should ascertain the context in which the behavior occurs. Finally, the nonspecificity of the term may result in a single-treatment approach with medications that have substantial side effects.[146] As with other BPSDs, agitation has been associated with caregiver depression and poor mental and physical health.[131,147]

Many standardized scales exist to measure behavioral disturbances. One of the most widely used scales is the Cohen-Mansfield Agitation Inventory. This instrument was constructed and tested for validity among nursing home residents and has since been validated in other settings.[148] Factor analysis revealed three categories: aggressive behavior (verbal aggression such as screaming and cursing or physical aggression such as hitting and scratching), physical nonaggressive behavior (pacing, hiding things, restlessness, wandering), and verbal nonaggressive behaviors (repeated requests for attention, complaining, interrupting).[149] In studies of people with dementia that use this scale, aggressive behaviors are more commonly found in men, specifically those with a premorbid history of aggression, greater cognitive impairment, and conflict with their caregiver.[150] Physical nonaggressive behaviors are associated with better physical health and greater cognitive impairment.[151] Verbal agitation is associated with female gender, social isolation, sensory impairment, pain, physical restraints, and functional impairment.[152]

Depending on the contributing etiologies of agitation, pharmacologic and nonpharmacologic treatment approaches should be considered. Nonpharmacologic interventions can be divided into three broad categories:[153]

- unmet needs intervention—conceptualizes the behavior as an underlying need
- learning and behavioral intervention—behavior leads to a consequence that reinforces continuation of the undesirable behavior
- environmental vulnerability and reduced stress thresholds intervention—a mismatch between the setting and the patient's ability to deal with it.

## Table 15. Causes Contributing to Agitation in Dementia

| Contributing Cause | Consideration | Treatment Approach |
|---|---|---|
| Physical symptom | Pain<br>Sleep disturbance | Analgesics<br>Behavior modification, sedative-hypnotic drugs |
| Psychological symptom | Depression | Antidepressant |
| Medical illness | Delirium<br>Seizure disorder<br>Constipation<br>Urinary retention<br>Psychosis<br>Dehydration<br>Infection | Evaluate predisposing causes<br>Treat underlying condition |
| Unmet need | Hunger<br>Social isolation<br>Soiled diaper | Attend to need |
| Sensory impairment | Vision loss<br>Hearing loss | Adaptive devices |
| Environment | Unfamiliar surroundings<br>Overstimulation<br>Understimulation | Modify environment |
| Medication/substance | Digoxin<br>Theophylline<br>Methylphenidate<br>Caffeine<br>Antipsychotic<br>Benzodiazepine | Decrease dosage or discontinue agent based on specific prognosis, goals of care, and risk benefit ratio |
| Underlying dementia | Alzheimer's disease<br>Vascular dementia<br>Lewy body dementia<br>Mixed dementia<br>Other | Evaluate severity of symptom and consider risk-benefit ratio of available treatments |

In a 2006 metaanalysis, the study's authors concluded that nonpharmacologic interventions that address unmet needs and behavioral issues can be effective. Because of the relationship between unmet needs and agitation, changes in behavior should prompt screening for elder mistreatment.[153]

Since the publication of the metaanalysis, several promising well-conducted nonpharmacologic treatment strategies have emerged as being helpful for agitation in people with dementia. A couple of small randomized controlled trials have demonstrated significant benefits in decreasing agitation with aromatherapy.[145] A family caregiver intervention of community-dwelling people with moderate dementia found substantial improvement in the most problematic behavior identified, including agitation; 67.5% improvement occurred in the intervention group versus 45.8% improvement in the no-treatment control ($P < .01$).[154] The intervention consisted of multiple home and telephone contacts performed by nurses and occupational therapists over 16 weeks, with the goal of identifying behavior triggers and training caregivers in strategies to modify the trigger and modify their reaction. Unfortunately, as with many nonpharmacologic interventions, the study's benefits appeared to wane over time. Lastly, a nursing home study implemented a patient-centered approach in which standard stimuli were introduced to people with moderate to severe dementia and agitation.[155] The stimuli included live social (a real baby, a dog, and one-on-one socializing), task (flower arranging and coloring), reading, listening to music, working (stamping envelopes, folding clothes, and sorting items), simulated social (a doll, plush animal, and robotic animal), manipulative (squeeze ball, activity pillow, building blocks, fabric book, wallet for men and purse for women, and puzzle), and usual care. The study demonstrated that any type of stimulus was preferable to standard nursing home care; the stimuli more effectively addressed physical agitation than verbal agitation, and live social stimuli was generally most effective.

Pharmacologic studies that examine the benefits of active drug therapy compared with placebo for the treatment of agitation fail to consider the numerous contributors to agitation and most often assume that a given symptom is related to the underlying neurodegenerative disease. Pharmacologic treatment should be considered only after a patient with dementia and his caregiver have undergone a thorough history to discern potential contributors to the agitation. This evaluation should be followed by a focused physical examination and relevant laboratory or radiologic studies. When the clinician is confident the agitation is related to the underlying dementia, the pharmacologic treatments described in this book may be considered.

As with treatment for psychosis and delusions, evidence suggests typical and atypical antipsychotics are modestly effective as agitation treatment for people with dementia, but they can cause significant side effects.[136-138] Additional agents that have been used for the treatment of agitation for dementia are displayed in **Table 16** and include antidepressants such as trazodone and SSRIs,[156-158] cholinesterase inhibitors,[48] NMDA receptor antagonists,[159] anxiolytics (ie, benzodiazepines),[160] as well as newer "older" agents such as dextromethorphan-quinidine.[161-163] The literature reports the effectiveness of these agents as mixed. Their use should be weighed

## Table 16. Pharmacologic Approaches to Treatment of Agitation in Dementia[165]

| Agent | Dosage (Starting/Maximal) | Evidence | Common Side Effects |
|---|---|---|---|
| **Atypical antipsychotics*** | See Table 14 | RCT | See Table 14 |
| **Atypical antidepressants** | | | |
| Trazodone | 25 mg-50 mg/200 mg per day | RCT | Sedation, postural hypotension |
| **SSRIs** | | | |
| Citalopram | 10 mg per day/20 mg per day | RCT | Nausea, insomnia, somnolence |
| **Benzodiazepines** | | | |
| Lorazepam | 0.25 mg twice daily/4 mg per day | RCT | Ataxia, sedation, falls, "paradoxical" agitation |
| **Cholinesterase inhibitors** | See Table 10 | RCT | See Table 10 |
| **NMDA receptor antagonists** | See Table 10 | RCT | See Table 10 |
| Dextromethorphan-quinidine[165] | 20 mg dextromethorphan and 10 mg quinidine twice daily after 1 week at once daily | | Prolonged QT, dizziness |

*NMDA, N-methyl-D-asparate; RCT, randomized controlled trial; SSRI, selective serotonin reuptake inhibitors. *The US Food and Drug Administration (FDA) added black box warnings to several medications commonly used by hospice and palliative care practitioners. Black box warnings are designed to highlight the potential for rare but serious medical complications such as stroke or myocardial infarction associated with the use of these drugs. Hospice and palliative care practitioners should be aware of these FDA black box warnings and the risk-benefit ratio of these medications and alternatives for individual patients. The short prognosis and critical importance of symptom relief for many hospice and palliative care patients may justify the use of these medications despite such risks.*

carefully against relative efficacy, adverse effects, and cost. One study of the use of tetrahydrocannabinol (THC; the psychoactive compound in marijuana) has been done, but the results did not show any improvement in symptoms; however, it was well-tolerated, which suggests further study is warranted.[164]

Geriatric treatment principles are paramount when considering use of pharmacologic agents to treat agitation in dementia, especially because patients with dementia have diminished cognitive and functional reserves. After an appropriate evaluation and treatment of any contributing conditions, healthcare providers should consider whether the agitation results in enough patient or caregiver distress to warrant treatment. If treatment is warranted, a non-pharmacologic approach should be considered first. If pharmacologic therapy is determined to be the appropriate next step, establish a clear treatment goal and consider discontinuing the medication if there is no discernable improvement within several weeks of therapy initiation. Considering the side-effect profile of currently available medications, begin with the lowest possible effective dosage and titrate upward slowly until the goal of therapy is achieved. Because BPSDs can change over time, consider lowering the dosage or discontinuing the therapy altogether to see whether the behavior recurs.

## Clinical Situation

### Lucja's Case Continues (Continued from page 69)

Four years after diagnosis Lucja is living in a nursing home. She is dependent in all of her IADLs, and although she is continent and can feed herself, she now requires assistance with bathing, dressing, and transferring. Two years ago memantine was added to her regimen because of a progressive decline in her cognition and functioning while on a cholinesterase inhibitor. Lucja recently developed aggressive behaviors, including screaming and hitting caregivers, and these behaviors have not responded to antidepressants and behavioral therapy. After risks and benefits were discussed with Pawel, she was started on quetiapine, an antipsychotic drug, and her condition has been stable for 6 months. Lucja has presented to the physician's office with worsening aggression, agitation, and social withdrawal during the past 2 weeks. Because of the change in her behaviors, her quetiapine dose was increased. Pawel is concerned that his mother may be discharged from the facility or sent to a behavioral unit and is requesting more sedating medications.

 This is a difficult time for all involved, but the most important intervention should be a careful history from the facility, including multiple shifts of caregivers, along with examination.

 Assessment of agitation requires a broad and thoughtful approach. Only after a comprehensive evaluation can agitation and aggression be considered the result of the underlying neurodegenerative process. Potential contributors to agitation and aggression include physical symptoms, sensory impairment, psychological symptoms, medical illness, medications, unmet needs, and environment.

Treatment with antipsychotic medications is not without concerns as previously described. Pawel's concern about his mother's placement should be addressed with staff, and careful adjustments should be made to her medications and care plans. Only after these interventions have failed should other options be considered, including more sedating drugs.

### The Case Continues

The clinical staff notes Lucja has poor appetite and difficulty sleeping. Cognitively she is oriented to person and place, recalls zero out of three words at 5 minutes, and has intact attention. Her vital signs are normal, but she has lost 7 pounds since her last appointment 1 month ago. On physical examination her right knee is swollen and painful with decreased range of motion. There is no evidence of fecal impaction or urinary retention. Laboratory measurements, including urinalysis, were negative. An X-ray of the knee revealed a moderate-sized effusion with chondrocalcinosis. Lucja was placed on a steroid taper with around-the-clock acetaminophen. Within a few days her pain decreased significantly, her appetite improved, she became more social, and her agitation resolved. This allowed the quetiapine dosage to be decreased to the previously prescribed level.

*Case continues on page 88*

## End-Stage Issues

As dementia progresses to the advanced stage, the affected person becomes dependent upon others for all of her care. At the end stage, people with dementia are bed bound, incontinent of stool and urine, develop difficulty handling secretions, and utter few if any intelligible words. This stage places patients at high risk for developing complications such as acute infection (urinary-tract, pneumonia), febrile episodes, swallowing difficulties (dysphagia, aspiration), injuries and trauma (hip or other bone fractures), and stroke.[7,37,38,166] Ideally, before the patient develops an acute event, healthcare providers and the patient's power of attorney should discuss treatment preferences to consider once a complication develops. *UNIPAC 6* outlines ethical principles to consider (beneficence, autonomy, nonmaleficence, justice) when making treatment decisions for vulnerable patients with limited life expectancy and describes a framework for considering these complex issues.

Conversations with families about end-stage issues remain particularly important because patients dying of dementia often receive suboptimal end-of-life care that includes poor symptom control, inappropriate procedures, and placement in restraints.[167] At the same time, hospice is underused for people dying from dementia[87,168] even though multiple studies document its benefits for patients and families.[169-172] A 2017 study using a goals of care decision aid improved end-of-life communication for nursing home residents with advanced dementia and enhanced palliative care plans while reducing hospital transfers.[173]

The goal of this section is to provide healthcare professionals with the medical knowledge to conduct a thoughtful and accurate dialogue with surrogates to help them weigh the burdens and benefits associated with medical therapies commonly used near end of life.

## Eating Difficulties

Dementia predisposes patients to eating and swallowing difficulties such as diminished reserve, apraxia, and dysphagia. Mealtime represents a stimulating experience that can overwhelm a person with dementia through visual, auditory, and olfactory sensory activation. When apraxia develops, a patient with dementia does not recognize food and forgets how to use utensils. Finger foods and large spoons can help. Also, cups should be small and not have handles. Finally, food should be served one course at a time, and there should not be too much food on the patient's plate nor too many objects on the table; items such as paper napkins can distract patients.

In the advanced stages of dementia, chewing food can take longer; frequently patients require help with swallowing in the form of cues such as verbal reminders, imitation of the process, or stroking the patient's throat or cheek. Neuromuscular problems in the pharyngeal musculature (eg, degenerative changes in corticobulbar tracts and cranial nerve nuclei) can lead to dysphagia and choking on liquids and solids.[174] Dysphagia usually develops gradually, progressing from occurrence with consumption of solids, then purées, and then liquids. If acute dysphagia develops, a thoughtful medical workup for reversible conditions should be performed.

Caloric intake in people with dementia often fails to meet metabolic requirements. As discussed previously, dysphagia may impede adequate oral intake. Other contributors to eating difficulties may include conditions associated with the mouth and gastrointestinal tract (eg, poor dentition, thrush, oral ulcers, delayed gastric emptying, fecal impaction, dry mouth); medication-related anorexia resulting from diuretics, beta blockers (with subsequent masking of hypoglycemia), digoxin, nonsteroidal antiinflammatory agents, cholinesterase inhibitors, and amiodarone; and unrecognized symptoms such as depression, pain, and nausea.[175,176] Because of poor oral intake, slow-hand feeding, which takes considerable time (often more than 1 hour per meal), often is required.

When weight loss occurs or oral intake diminishes to an unacceptable level (often during an acute event such as pneumonia), the issue of feeding tube use often arises. Feeding tube placement for people with advanced dementia continued to increase despite the lack of literature supporting its use; however, a 2016 study shows decreased use for the first time.[177-180] The use of feeding tubes in patients with advanced dementia from 2000 to 2014 has declined from 11.7% to 5.7%. However, African American residents (17.5%) continue to receive more tube feeding than white residents (3.1%).[180] Reasons frequently cited for feeding tube placement include decreased mortality and aspiration, improved nutritional and functional status, and healing of pressure ulcers.[181] Although no randomized controlled trials exist that compare hand feeding with tube feeding for end-stage patients with dementia, cohort and cross-sectional studies provide convincing evidence that tube feeding does not improve patient outcomes.[182] Mortality is high with or without feeding tube placement, with 30-day mortality averaging about 20%, 6-month mortality at 50%, and a median survival of 56 days.[177,183,184] Aspiration often continues after feeding tube placement, and many patients develop new aspiration after the tube is placed.[185] At the same time, feeding tube placement detracts from patient-focused care and is associated with frequent complications requiring transfer back to an acute-care hospital for additional interventions.[177] No studies published to date have assessed the impact on QOL of a feeding tube compared with slow-hand feeding. Many of the reasons cited for feeding tube placement are not supported by the evidence, and the burden of the intervention may outweigh the benefits of continued slow-hand feeding. The American Geriatric Society position statement on the use of feeding tubes in advanced dementia was published in 2014. This position statement documents the real harms attributable to feeding tubes, which include increased agitation, greater use of physical and chemical restraints, as well as burdensome transitions of care due to tube-related complications and the development of new pressure ulcers.[186]

More efforts now focus on addressing goals of care related to feeding decisions before the question of a feeding tube arises. One approach has been to use a video decision support tool to facilitate advance care planning in cognitively intact people in the event that dementia develops and progresses to the advanced stage.[187] Compared with a verbal description, a video depiction was more likely to be associated with goals of care in advanced dementia that focus on comfort. Moreover, participants who watched the video had more stable preferences over time. Another approach currently being researched assesses the usefulness of a decisional support tool to facilitate advance care planning with surrogates regarding tube feeding in nursing home residents with advanced dementia.

### Infection Treatment

Invariably a person with advanced dementia develops an infectious complication, usually a urinary-tract infection or pneumonia. Work by Teno and others continues to study the outcome of burdensome transitions on patients with advanced dementia. These studies suggest that the outcome is the same whether treatment occurs in the nursing home or the hospital. These studies also indicate that the first hospitalization for nursing home residents with advanced cognitive impairment should include reconsideration of the goals of care and the appropriateness of continued hospitalizations.[188] In addition, Dufour and colleagues found that treatment of urinary tract infection in patients with advanced dementia did not alter survival.[189] One earlier study found an in-hospital mortality of almost 20% in patients with advanced dementia receiving antibiotics, with a 6-month mortality rate of more than 50%.[38] During hospitalization, patients undergo many procedures that are reported to be painful, including daily blood draws, arterial blood-gas measurement, and intravenous (IV)-line placement. In addition, hospitalized patients with dementia remain at high risk for being placed in restraints to receive IV antibiotics and oxygen therapy.[38,190] Given these facts, it is not surprising that many dementia experts recommend that people with advanced dementia who have infectious complications not be hospitalized, as is practiced in other countries.[191] Moreover, compared with good palliative care (including antipyretics, analgesics, and oxygen), antibiotics do not improve patients' comfort, although they have been shown to improve survival for patients with advanced dementia and pneumonia.[192,193]

## Hip Fractures

Hip fractures commonly occur in older adults with or without cognitive impairment. Bed-bound patients remain at risk for hip fracture, which can occur either during routine care (chair transfers, bathing, or changing soiled diapers) or spontaneously. The decision of whether to surgically repair a hip fracture in a bed-bound patient with severe cognitive impairment is challenging and requires consideration of the risks associated with hospitalization and surgical repair compared with palliative and hospice care. Surgery can be considered palliative because pain is likely to be less severe after the repair. The in-hospital mortality rate for fractured hip repair in patients with advanced dementia is relatively low (about 5%), but the 6-month mortality rate remains high (more than 50%).[38] People with dementia who have a hip fracture and who undergo surgical repair experience undertreated pain. In fact, 76% of patients with advanced dementia who were hospitalized for surgical repair did not receive a standing analgesic agent, according to two studies.[194,195]

The nonsurgical palliative approach to hip fractures for patients with end-stage dementia focuses on symptom management and prevention of complications. The predominant physical symptom after a hip fracture, particularly during routine care, is pain. As such, patients with hip fracture should not only receive adequate analgesia throughout the day to maintain comfort but also premedication before repositioning, transferring, and performing daily care activities such as dressing and bathing. Often, when opioids are required to adequately control a patient's pain, increased sedation may occur. Ultimately the risk-benefit ratio of opioid use must be considered in the context of the patient's QOL, goals of care, and limited life expectancy. One of the most common complications of hip fractures is the development of skin breakdown, which can occur despite the most rigorous preventive care, including repositioning frequently, getting patients out of bed, and optimizing nutrition. Given the poor prognosis of patients with hip fracture who have end-stage dementia, hospice referral should be considered and discussed with the patient's power of attorney independent of a decision about surgical repair.

### Lucja's Case Continues (Continued from page 84)

Seven years after diagnosis, Lucja is wheelchair bound. She is incontinent of stool and urine and utters 6 to 10 intelligible words a day. During the past month, she has required more assistance with feeding and is pocketing food in her mouth. She recently was admitted for pneumonia, has developed a stage 2 sacral pressure ulcer, and has lost 15 pounds within the last 6 months. Pawel is concerned about Lucja's eating and comes in to discuss feeding tube placement as well as goals of care. Family medical history reveals that Lucja's sister had a feeding tube placed after a cerebrovascular accident. Further discussions with Pawel were held to educate him on the expectations of careful hand feeding as well as gastrostomy tube placement.

 Many conditions may contribute to declines in oral intake. Mouth-related issues include dryness, thrush, ulcers, and poor dentition. Delayed gastric emptying, constipation, gastroesophageal reflux, and fecal impaction also may be associated with poor oral intake. Medications frequently associated with anorexia include digoxin, beta blockers, diuretics, and amiodarone. Finally, unrecognized symptoms such as pain, shortness of breath, agitation, depression, and nausea may contribute to poor intake.

 Caregivers are unaware that feeding tubes frequently are placed in people with end-stage dementia despite the fact that the data suggest little or no role for the reasons frequently cited. Feeding tubes have not been shown to decrease mortality or the rates of aspiration pneumonia. They also have not been shown to improve functional status, pressure-ulcer healing, or nutritional status. Feeding tubes have not been shown to decrease the rate of hospitalization and, in fact, may increase risk because of complications associated with the placement and use of the tube.

 Careful and thoughtful discussions occur to elicit goals of care, and information is provided about putting plans into place for palliating discomfort and avoiding burdensome hospitalizations for future infections. End-stage dementia from progressive neurodegeneration is associated with apraxia, dysphagia, and immobility that put people at high risk for medical complications. Common complications of end-stage dementia include pressure sores, infections (pneumonia and urinary tract), hip fractures, and malnutrition.

 A hospice service should be explained and offered for continuing care. Pawel clearly cares for his mother, and answering his questions and concerns in an empathetic manner is most helpful.

*Case continues on page 93*

## Treatment of Comorbid Conditions

Several papers on inappropriate prescription of medication for older adult populations have been published. At the same time, disease-specific guidelines on appropriate pharmacotherapy continue to be created and revised. People with dementia have multiple morbidities that require numerous medications to comply with "current recommendations." Also, people with dementia take prescription and nonprescription drugs for their underlying neurodegenerative disease. As a result, these patients may be on a plethora of medications, many of which can interact and have additive side effects. For example, patients on cholinesterase inhibitors who develop urinary incontinence are likely to be placed on anticholinergics, which may lead to nausea and dry mouth, predisposing them to dehydration.

One approach to minimizing polypharmacy is to prioritize existing medications and consider discontinuing therapies that may no longer be providing clinical benefit consistent with the goals of care. To date, little attention has been given to determining whether otherwise appropriate therapy should be discontinued for people nearing the end of life.[196] One frequently cited article suggests that a decision-making model should take into account remaining life expectancy, time until benefit is derived, goals of care, and treatment targets (ie, primary and secondary prevention and symptom control).[197] Using such an approach, healthcare providers can engage patients (when appropriate) and families in shared decision making about starting, stopping, or continuing therapy.[198]

Unfortunately, few studies are available to guide clinicians on which medications are least likely to provide clinically relevant benefits. This lack of information poses particular challenges when a medication may be offering some symptomatic benefit and the patient cannot relate their experience. It is important to advise families about treatments that they are absolutely convinced are helping the patient, and to help them to understand that hospice is not giving up on or denying pharmacologic therapy.

## Hospice

Research suggests that patients dying of dementia receive suboptimal end-of-life care that includes poor symptom control and overly aggressive treatments. Despite research suggesting little or no benefit, many patients with end-stage dementia die with feeding tubes in place and undergo mechanical ventilation.[178,179] Compared with patients dying of cancer in nursing homes, dying patients with dementia are more likely to undergo bloodwork and be restrained.[167] Families may opt for extensive diagnostic workups, aggressive treatment of coexisting medical conditions, transfer to an acute-care facility with any change in condition, and cardiopulmonary resuscitation in the event of an arrest, which detracts from a palliative approach and has not been shown to prolong survival.[199] People with dementia living in nursing homes, hospitals, and within communities are at risk for inadequate pain management. In one study, people with cognitive impairment who underwent hip surgery were given one-third the amount of opioid analgesic administered to cognitively intact patients.[194,195] Compared with cognitively intact nursing home residents in pain, cognitively impaired nursing home residents in pain were much less likely to receive analgesia.[94] Among community-dwelling people with dementia who could still report their pain experience, half of those who reported pain "on an average day" were not taking an analgesic.[200]

Many healthcare providers and families believe hospice care is the most appropriate care near the end of life.[77] Moreover, no effective treatment of dementia exists, and patients exhibit considerable physical symptoms and self-care needs at the end of life.[172] At the same time, caregivers experience a substantial burden and can benefit from additional support.[201] Despite the apparent need and the belief that hospice care is appropriate, a minority of patients—fewer than 10%—with advanced dementia die with the benefits of hospice services.[87]

Hospice eligibility guidelines (see Table 11) generally specify that a patient with dementia must maintain substantial functional limitations (Functional Assessment Stage 7 or beyond, depending on Medicare Administrative Contractor: bed bound, uttering few words, and requiring assistance with ambulation) and present with disease complications (eg, aspiration pneumonia, upper urinary-tract infection, septicemia, multiple decubitus ulcers), recurrent fever despite antibiotics, and inability to take in sufficient fluids and food to sustain life.[83] The Functional Assessment Staging Scale (FAST) has the following limitations[93]:

- It was not developed to predict life expectancy.
- It presents functional loss as an ordinal progression that is not necessarily the way in which the disease progresses.
- It is not derived from empirical data. In fact, one study found that hospice guidelines were better at predicting who would *not* die within 6 months than who would die.[202]

Although many studies support the benefits of hospice care for patients with cancer, few studies have been conducted among people with dementia. One study of nursing home residents, in which a majority were dying as a result of dementia, found that those enrolled in hospice were twice as likely as nonhospice enrollees to receive regular treatment for pain.[203] Similarly, a nursing home study found that people dying with dementia on hospice were more likely to receive scheduled opioids for pain and directed therapies for dyspnea (oxygen, opioids, scopolamine, and hyoscamine); in addition, caregivers reported fewer unmet needs during the last 7 days of life compared with those who were not enrolled in hospice.[204] In another study of community-dwelling older adults with dementia who were dying, hospice enrollees were significantly more likely than nonenrollees to die in their location of choice—almost always at home—and less likely to die in a hospital. Caregivers of enrollees also were more likely to report care to be excellent or very good compared with caregivers of nonenrollees. However, the mean pain scores of hospice enrollees and nonenrollees were not significantly different, and on average caregivers for both groups reported the patient's pain at a moderate or higher intensity during the last 2 weeks of life.[203] On the whole, hospice improves the care of people dying with dementia, but more work is needed to better understand the assessment and treatment of physical symptoms that occur near the end of life for patients across care settings, including the community, nursing homes, and hospitals. Another scenario arises when caring for people with dementia—families often request hospice services for a loved one with advanced disease that is not yet severe enough to meet hospice eligibility criteria if only the FAST scale is used. A patient who is bed bound and incontinent with a recent pneumonia and can still utter more than six intelligible words per day is an example of such a patient. In such cases in which hospice admission is agreed upon, it is imperative for hospice and palliative care providers to document the reasons a patient's prognosis is shorter than 6 months (eg, recurrent aspiration pneumonia, accelerated weight loss, or recent stroke). Throughout the hospice course it is necessary that the team continue to document disease progression, and at recertification periods prognosis data must be reiterated, preferably with objective documented evidence of decline (eg, number of pneumonia episodes, number of centimeters of decreased triceps fold thickness, increased dependency with feeding).

## Issues for Caregivers

Compared with other chronic, disabling, life-limiting conditions, caring for a person with AD or related dementia poses unique stressors and challenges. With AD, the caregiver role usually lasts for many years and changes over time as the disease progresses. In addition to cognitive losses (eg, short-term memory, orientation, language difficulties, executive functioning), patients often develop personality changes and exhibit challenging behaviors such as agitation and aggression, loud vocalizations, and wandering. Over time, people with dementia require greater supervision during self-care activities and throughout the day and night to ensure adequate safety. Compared with other caregivers, those who care for people with dementia must provide greater assistance when transferring loved ones in and out of bed and with dressing, bathing, toileting, and changing incontinence products.[19] Given these additional needs, caregivers of people with dementia report greater physical and emotional strain, take fewer vacations, have fewer hobbies, spend less time with other family members, and have more work-related difficulties such as having to reduce hours to part time, turn down promotions, and lose job benefits compared with caregivers of physically impaired older adults.[205]

Although caregiving provides many altruistic benefits for the caregiver, it comes at a considerable cost, particularly when caring for those with dementia. Caregivers of people with dementia have higher rates of depression and anxiety, and female caregivers report higher levels of depression and anxiety compared with male caregivers.[206-208] At the same time, caregivers are less likely to participate in preventive health behaviors and report mental and physical health problems that arise from their caregiving.[205,206] Caregivers who reported mental and emotional strain had a 63% higher mortality risk than controls who did not report mental or emotional strain.[209] Given the increased strain on caregivers and the underlying vulnerability of people with dementia, it is not surprising that dementia is a risk factor for the mistreatment of older adults.

A recent study suggests that care provided through hospice enrollment improves the consequences of unrelieved psychological distress such as depression, anxiety, and perceived severity of pain. Care provided through hospice enrollment also helped improve physical symptoms that affect health and QOL; these symptoms can impair decision making, impact the relationship with the care recipient, and increase the probability of morbidity, mortality, and suicide. Effective strategies to ameliorate psychological distress, particularly in the setting of caregiving for family members with AD, are likely to have a profound impact on the end-of-life experiences of these patients and their family members. Hospice care may serve as a model to deliver such interventions and thereby support caregivers in this final phase of caring for loved ones with AD.[210]

Caregivers face many difficult decisions as dementia progresses for their loved one. These decisions often come at a substantial cost for both themselves and the patient and may include taking over the patient's finances, taking away their car keys, and placing them in a nursing home. Certain patient and caregiver characteristics have been found to increase risk for nursing home placement for people with dementia.[211,212] Patient characteristics included being Caucasian, living alone, having greater functional and cognitive impairment, and exhibiting difficult behaviors. Caregiver characteristics included being older than 65 years and reporting a greater burden. Caregivers who reported that providing help to their relative made them feel useful, appreciated, and important were significantly less likely to place their relative in a long-term-care facility. At the same time, caregivers who chose long-term care for their loved one did not report a decrease in depressive or anxiety symptoms; these effects were most pronounced among caregivers who were spouses, visited the patient more frequently, and reported less satisfaction with the help they received from others.

Many intervention studies have been designed to decrease caregiver burden and depression. These interventions focused on both the patient with dementia (eg, reducing care-recipient behaviors and dependency) and the patient's caregiver (eg, providing knowledge about caregiving and the relationship with the care recipient, available community resources and support, coping with and resolving feelings of depression and anxiety). Research suggests that the interventions that have the largest impact and greatest success take the caregiver's strengths and abilities into account, target multiple domains, and focus on both members of the dyad (ie, the patient with dementia and the caregiver).[213,214] A randomized, controlled, and structured multicomponent intervention found the intervention arm was associated with lower rates of depression and greater improvement in QOL for Hispanic, Caucasian, and African American caregivers.[215] Caregiver health also improved; the intervention group reported better self-rated health, sleep, mood improvement, and physical improvement compared with the control group.[216] Despite these findings, the effect size of caregiver interventions may be smaller for those who care for people with dementia compared with other caregivers.[217] Recent trials of the Internet intervention "Mastery over Dementia" for family caregivers of people with dementia suggest a reduction of symptoms of depression and anxiety. These findings are promising because future generations will have more Internet access.[218] Local branches of the Alzheimer's Association can provide caregivers with access to support groups and helpful educational courses. The Alzheimer's Association website, www.alz.org, offers a tremendous amount of educational material for caregivers.

The end-of-life and bereavement experience for caregivers of people with dementia who are living at home has been characterized.[201] Fifty percent of caregivers report spending 46 hours weekly helping their relative with ADLs and IADLs. More than 50% of caregivers reported feeling "on duty" 24 hours a day to perform their caregiving role. Before their relative's death, 43% of caregivers had substantial depressive symptoms, which declined significantly 3 months after the patient's death and within 1 year were significantly lower than when they acted as a caregiver. Complicated grief was more common among caregivers who had high levels of depressive symptoms and burden before their relative's death than in those who reported positive features of caregiving and who cared for relatives with greater cognitive impairment.[219]

See *UNIPAC 2* for more information about caregivers.

## Clinical Situation

### Lucja's Case Concludes (Continued from page 88)

Lucja now eats by slow hand feeding with cues, is taking in minimal calories, and continues to lose weight. All of her medications, including donepezil, and memantine have been discontinued. She is now bed bound and completely dependent in all ADLs. She develops occasional periods of restlessness and fevers that respond to acetaminophen.

After much discussion, Lucja is enrolled in a hospice program and dies peacefully in the nursing home 4 months after hospice enrollment.

The hospice eligibility criteria for dementia require the disease to be advanced enough to result in substantial functional limitations and severe enough to be associated with medical complications. From a functional standpoint, the patient must be unable to walk, dress, or bathe without assistance; have urinary and fecal incontinence; and be unable to speak six different intelligible words in a day. At least one medical complication should occur during the previous 6 months and include aspiration pneumonia, pyelonephritis, septicemia, multiple stage 3 or stage 4 pressure sores, fever despite antibiotics, or weight loss exceeding 10% of body weight.

For people with a primary diagnosis of dementia, the hospice benefit provides patient and caregiver outcomes that are superior to routine care. Patients in hospice are more likely to die at home and are more likely to be prescribed medications for pain. Caregivers report higher satisfaction with care and receive additional support. Studies have not examined whether hospice enrollment for people with dementia is associated with a longer life expectancy.

# References

1. Lanctot KL, Herrmann N, Rothenburg L, Eryavec G. Behavioral correlates of GABAergic disruption in Alzheimer's disease. *Int Psychogeriatr.* 2007;19(1):151-158.

2. McKee AC, Cantu RC, Nowinski CJ, et al. Chronic traumatic encephalopathy in athletes: progressive tauopathy after repetitive head injury. *J Neuropathol Exp Neurol.* 2009;68(7):709-735.

3. Petersen RC, Smith G, Kokmen E, Ivnik RJ, Tangalos EG. Memory function in normal aging. *Neurology.* 1992;42(2):396-401.

4. Busse A, Angermeyer MC, Riedel-Heller SG. Progression of mild cognitive impairment to dementia: a challenge to current thinking. *Br J Psychiatry.* 2006;189:399-404.

5. Barker WW, Luis CA, Kashuba A, et al. Relative frequencies of Alzheimer disease, Lewy body, vascular and frontotemporal dementia, and hippocampal sclerosis in the State of Florida Brain Bank. *Alzheimer Dis Assoc Disord.* 2002;16(4):203-212.

6. Blennow K, de Leon MJ, Zetterberg H. Alzheimer's disease. *Lancet.* 2006;368(9533):387-403.

7. Morris JC, McKeel DW, Jr., Fulling K, Torack RM, Berg L. Validation of clinical diagnostic criteria for Alzheimer's disease. *Ann Neurol.* 1988;24(1):17-22.

8. McKhann G, Drachman D, Folstein M, Katzman R, Price D, Stadlan EM. Clinical diagnosis of Alzheimer's disease: report of the NINCDS-ADRDA Work Group under the auspices of Department of Health and Human Services Task Force on Alzheimer's Disease. *Neurology.* 1984;34(7):939-944.

9. Jost BC, Grossberg GT. The evolution of psychiatric symptoms in Alzheimer's disease: a natural history study. *J Am Geriatr Soc.* 1996;44(9):1078-1081.

10. Reitz C, Brayne C, Mayeux R. Epidemiology of Alzheimer disease. *Nat Rev Neurol.* 2011;7(3):137-152.

11. Jack CR, Jr., Knopman DS, Jagust WJ, et al. Hypothetical model of dynamic biomarkers of the Alzheimer's pathological cascade. *Lancet Neurol.* 2010;9(1):119-128.

12. Geldmacher DS, Whitehouse PJ. Evaluation of dementia. *N Engl J Med.* 1996;335(5):330-336.

13. Bowler JV. Vascular cognitive impairment. *J Neurol Neurosurg Psychiatry.* 1996;76:35-44.

14. Kirshner HS. Vascular dementia: a review of recent evidence for prevention and treatment. *Curr Neurol Neurosci Rep.* 2009;9(6):437-442.

15. Snowdon DA, Greiner LH, Mortimer JA, Riley KP, Greiner PA, Markesbery WR. Brain infarction and the clinical expression of Alzheimer disease. The Nun Study. *JAMA.* 1997;277(10):813-817.

16. McKeith IG, Dickson DW, Lowe J, et al. Diagnosis and management of dementia with Lewy bodies: third report of the DLB Consortium. *Neurology.* 2005;65(12):1863-1872.

17. Dodel R, Csoti I, Ebersbach G, et al. Lewy body dementia and Parkinson's disease with dementia. *J Neurol.* 2008;255 Suppl 5:39-47.

18. Evans DA, Scherr PA, Smith LA, Albert MS, Funkenstein HH. The east Boston Alzheimer's Disease Registry. *Aging (Milano).* 1990;2(3):298-302.

19. 2016 Alzheimer's disease facts and figures. *Alzheimers Dement.* 2016;12(4):459-509.

20. Bynum JP, Rabins PV, Weller W, Niefeld M, Anderson GF, Wu AW. The relationship between a dementia diagnosis, chronic illness, medicare expenditures, and hospital use. *J Am Geriatr Soc.* 2004;52(2):187-194.

21. McCarthy M, Addington-Hall J, Altmann D. The experience of dying with dementia: a retrospective study. *Int J Geriatr Psychiatry.* 1997;12(3):404-409.

22. Wolfson C, Wolfson DB, Asgharian M, et al. A reevaluation of the duration of survival after the onset of dementia. *N Engl J Med.* 2001;344(15):1111-1116.

23. Walsh JS, Welch HG, Larson EB. Survival of outpatients with Alzheimer-type dementia. *Ann Intern Med.* 1990;113(6):429-434.

24. Ganguli M, Dodge HH, Shen C, Pandav RS, DeKosky ST. Alzheimer disease and mortality: a 15-year epidemiological study. *Arch Neurol.* 2005;62(5):779-784.

25. Waring SC, Doody RS, Pavlik VN, Massman PJ, Chan W. Survival among patients with dementia from a large multi-ethnic population. *Alzheimer Dis Assoc Disord.* 2005;19(4):178-183.

26. Brookmeyer R, Corrada MM, Curriero FC, Kawas C. Survival following a diagnosis of Alzheimer disease. *Arch Neurol.* 2002;59(11):1764-1767.

27. Larson EB, Shadlen MF, Wang L, et al. Survival after initial diagnosis of Alzheimer disease. *Ann Intern Med.* 2004;140(7):501-509.

28. Helzner EP, Scarmeas N, Cosentino S, Tang MX, Schupf N, Stern Y. Survival in Alzheimer disease: a multiethnic, population-based study of incident cases. *Neurology.* 2008;71(19):1489-1495.

29. Xie J, Brayne C, Matthews FE. Survival times in people with dementia: analysis from population based cohort study with 14 year follow-up. *BMJ.* 2008;336(7638):258-262.

30. Rait G, Walters K, Bottomley C, Petersen I, Iliffe S, Nazareth I. Survival of people with clinical diagnosis of dementia in primary care: cohort study. *BMJ.* 2010;341:c3584.

31. Lunney JR, Lynn J, Foley DJ, Lipson S, Guralnik JM. Patterns of functional decline at the end of life. *JAMA.* 2003;289(18):2387-2392.

32. Helmes E, Merskey H, Fox H, Fry RN, Bowler JV, Hachinski VC. Patterns of deterioration in senile dementia of the Alzheimer type. *Arch Neurol.* 1995;52(3):306-310.

33. Sands LP, Yaffe K, Lui LY, Stewart A, Eng C, Covinsky K. The effects of acute illness on ADL decline over 1 year in frail older adults with and without cognitive impairment. *J Gerontol A Biol Sci Med Sci.* 2002;57(7):M449-454.

34. Sands LP, Yaffe K, Covinsky K, et al. Cognitive screening predicts magnitude of functional recovery from admission to 3 months after discharge in hospitalized elders. *J Gerontol A Biol Sci Med Sci.* 2003;58(1):37-45.

35. Kammoun S, Gold G, Bouras C, et al. Immediate causes of death of demented and non-demented elderly. *Acta Neurol Scand Suppl.* 2000;176:96-99.

36. Burns A, Jacoby R, Luthert P, Levy R. Cause of death in Alzheimer's disease. *Age Ageing.* 1990;19(5):341-344.

37. Mitchell SL, Teno JM, Kiely DK, et al. The clinical course of advanced dementia. *N Engl J Med.* 2009;361(16):1529-1538.

38. Morrison RS, Siu AL. Survival in end-stage dementia following acute illness. *JAMA.* 2000;284(1):47-52.

39. Hanyu H, Sato T, Hirao K, Kanetaka H, Sakurai H, Iwamoto T. Differences in clinical course between dementia with Lewy bodies and Alzheimer's disease. *Eur J Neurol.* 2009;16(2):212-217.

40. Hurley AC, Volicer L. Alzheimer Disease: "It's okay, Mama, if you want to go, it's okay". *JAMA.* 2002;288(18):2324-2331.

41. Brauner DJ, Muir JC, Sachs GA. Treating nondementia illnesses in patients with dementia. *JAMA.* 2000;283(24):3230-3235.

42. Shinotoh H, Fukushi K, Nagatsuka S, et al. The amygdala and Alzheimer's disease: positron emission tomographic study of the cholinergic system. *Ann NY Acad Sci.* 2003;985:411-419.

43. Tariot PN, Federoff HJ. Current treatment for Alzheimer disease and future prospects. *Alzheimer Dis Assoc Disord.* 2003;17 Suppl 4:S105-113.

44. Winblad B, Engedal K, Soininen H, et al. A 1-year, randomized, placebo-controlled study of donepezil in patients with mild to moderate AD. *Neurology.* 2001;57(3):489-495.

45. Farlow M, Anand R, Messina J, Jr., Hartman R, Veach J. A 52-week study of the efficacy of rivastigmine in patients with mild to moderately severe Alzheimer's disease. *Eur Neurol.* 2000;44(4):236-241.

46. Raskind MA, Peskind ER, Wessel T, Yuan W. Galantamine in AD: A 6-month randomized, placebo-controlled trial with a 6-month extension. The Galantamine USA-1 Study Group. *Neurology*. 2000;54(12):2261-2268.

47. Mohs RC, Doody RS, Morris JC, et al. A 1-year, placebo-controlled preservation of function survival study of donepezil in AD patients. *Neurology*. 2001;57(3):481-488.

48. Trinh NH, Hoblyn J, Mohanty S, Yaffe K. Efficacy of cholinesterase inhibitors in the treatment of neuropsychiatric symptoms and functional impairment in Alzheimer disease: a meta-analysis. *JAMA*. 2003;289(2):210-216.

49. Katz IR, Jeste DV, Mintzer JE, Clyde C, Napolitano J, Brecher M. Comparison of risperidone and placebo for psychosis and behavioral disturbances associated with dementia: a randomized, double-blind trial. Risperidone Study Group. *J Clin Psychiatry*. 1999;60(2):107-115.

50. Howard RJ, Juszczak E, Ballard CG, et al. Donepezil for the treatment of agitation in Alzheimer's disease. *N Engl J Med*. 2007;357(14):1382-1392.

51. O'Regan J, Lanctot KL, Mazereeuw G, Herrmann N. Cholinesterase inhibitor discontinuation in patients with Alzheimer's disease: a meta-analysis of randomized controlled trials. *J Clin Psychiatry*. 2015;76(11):e1424-1431.

52. Becker M, Andel R, Rohrer L, Banks SM. The effect of cholinesterase inhibitors on risk of nursing home placement among medicaid beneficiaries with dementia. *Alzheimer Dis Assoc Disord*. 2006;20(3):147-152.

53. Geldmacher DS, Provenzano G, McRae T, Mastey V, Ieni JR. Donepezil is associated with delayed nursing home placement in patients with Alzheimer's disease. *J Am Geriatr Soc*. 2003;51(7):937-944.

54. Winblad B, Kilander L, Eriksson S, et al. Donepezil in patients with severe Alzheimer's disease: double-blind, parallel-group, placebo-controlled study. *Lancet*. 2006;367(9516):1057-1065.

55. Feldman H, Gauthier S, Hecker J, Vellas B, Subbiah P, Whalen E. A 24-week, randomized, double-blind study of donepezil in moderate to severe Alzheimer's disease. *Neurology*. 2001;57(4):613-620.

56. Farlow MR, Salloway S, Tariot PN, et al. Effectiveness and tolerability of high-dose (23 mg/d) versus standard-dose (10 mg/d) donepezil in moderate to severe Alzheimer's disease: a 24-week, randomized, double-blind study. *Clin Ther*. 2010;32(7):1234-1251.

57. Shega JW, Ellner L, Lau DT, Maxwell TL. Cholinesterase inhibitor and N-methyl-D-aspartic acid receptor antagonist use in older adults with end-stage dementia: a survey of hospice medical directors. *J Palliat Med*. 2009;12(9):779-783.

58. Raina P, Santaguida P, Ismaila A, et al. Effectiveness of cholinesterase inhibitors and memantine for treating dementia: evidence review for a clinical practice guideline. *Ann Intern Med*. 2008;148(5):379-397.

59. McKeith I, Del Ser T, Spano P, et al. Efficacy of rivastigmine in dementia with Lewy bodies: a randomised, double-blind, placebo-controlled international study. *Lancet*. 2000;356(9247):2031-2036.

60. Roman GC, Wilkinson DG, Doody RS, Black SE, Salloway SP, Schindler RJ. Donepezil in vascular dementia: combined analysis of two large-scale clinical trials. *Dement Geriatr Cogn Disord*. 2005;20(6):338-344.

61. Emre M, Aarsland D, Albanese A, et al. Rivastigmine for dementia associated with Parkinson's disease. *N Engl J Med*. 2004;351(24):2509-2518.

62. Boot BP. Comprehensive treatment of dementia with Lewy bodies. *Alzheimers Res Ther*. 2015;7(1):45.

63. Courtney C, Farrell D, Gray R, et al. Long-term donepezil treatment in 565 patients with Alzheimer's disease (AD2000): randomised double-blind trial. *Lancet*. 2004;363(9427):2105-2115.

64. Danysz W, Parsons CG, Mobius HJ, Stoffler A, Quack G. Neuroprotective and symptomatological action of memantine relevant for Alzheimer's disease—a unified glutamatergic hypothesis on the mechanism of action. *Neurotox Res*. 2000;2(2-3):85-97.

65. Rogawski MA, Wenk GL. The neuropharmacological basis for the use of memantine in the treatment of Alzheimer's disease. *CNS Drug Rev.* 2003;9(3):275-308.

66. Reisberg B, Doody R, Stoffler A, Schmitt F, Ferris S, Mobius HJ. Memantine in moderate-to-severe Alzheimer's disease. *N Engl J Med.* 2003;348(14):1333-1341.

67. Tariot PN, Farlow MR, Grossberg GT, Graham SM, McDonald S, Gergel I. Memantine treatment in patients with moderate to severe Alzheimer disease already receiving donepezil: a randomized controlled trial. *JAMA.* 2004;291(3):317-324.

68. Howard R, McShane R, Lindesay J, et al. Donepezil and memantine for moderate-to-severe Alzheimer's disease. *N Engl J Med.* 2012;366(10):893-903.

69. Emre M, Tsolaki M, Bonuccelli U, et al. Memantine for patients with Parkinson's disease dementia or dementia with Lewy bodies: a randomised, double-blind, placebo-controlled trial. *Lancet Neurol.* 2010;9(10):969-977.

70. Buschert V, Bokde AL, Hampel H. Cognitive intervention in Alzheimer disease. *Nature reviews Neurology.* 2010;6(9):508-517.

71. Davis RN, Massman PJ, Doody RS. Cognitive intervention in Alzheimer disease: a randomized placebo-controlled study. *Alzheimer Dis Assoc Disord.* 2001;15(1):1-9.

72. Bassuk SS, Glass TA, Berkman LF. Social disengagement and incident cognitive decline in community-dwelling elderly persons. *Ann Intern Med.* 1999;131(3):165-173.

73. Koh K, Ray R, Lee J, Nair A, Ho T, Ang PC. Dementia in elderly patients: can the 3R mental stimulation programme improve mental status? *Age Ageing.* 1994;23(3):195-199.

74. Teri L, Gibbons LE, McCurry SM, et al. Exercise plus behavioral management in patients with Alzheimer disease: a randomized controlled trial. *JAMA.* 2003;290(15):2015-2022.

75. Potter R, Ellard D, Rees K, Thorogood M. A systematic review of the effects of physical activity on physical functioning, quality of life and depression in older people with dementia. *Int J Geriatr Psychiatry.* 2011.

76. Diesfeldt HF, van Houte LR, Moerkens RM. Duration of survival in senile dementia. *Acta Psychiatr Scand.* 1986;73(4):366-371.

77. Hanrahan P, Luchins DJ. Access to hospice programs in end-stage dementia: a national survey of hospice programs. *J Am Geriatr Soc.* 1995;43(1):56-59.

78. Doberman DJ, Yasar S, Durso SC. Would you refer this patient to hospice? An evaluation of tools for determining life expectancy in end-stage dementia. *J Palliat Med.* 2007;10(6):1410-1419.

79. Christakis NA, Escarce JJ. Survival of Medicare patients after enrollment in hospice programs. *N Engl J Med.* 1996;335(3):172-178.

80. Schonwetter RS, Han B, Small BJ, Martin B, Tope K, Haley WE. Predictors of six-month survival among patients with dementia: an evaluation of hospice Medicare guidelines. *Am J Hosp Palliat Care.* 2003;20(2):105-113.

81. Hanrahan P, Raymond M, McGowan E, Luchins DJ. Criteria for enrolling dementia patients in hospice: a replication. *Am J Hosp Palliat Care.* 1999;16(1):395-400.

82. Mitchell SL, Kiely DK, Hamel MB, Park PS, Morris JN, Fries BE. Estimating prognosis for nursing home residents with advanced dementia. *JAMA.* 2004;291(22):2734-2740.

83. Stuart B. The NHO Medical Guidelines for Non-Cancer Disease and local medical review policy: hospice access for patients with diseases other than cancer. *Hosp J.* 1999;14(3-4):139-154.

84. Centers for Medicare and Medicaid Services, US Department of Health and Human Services. Local Coverage Determinations (LCDs) by Contractor Index. https://www.cms.gov/medicare-coverage-database/indexes/lcd-contractor-index.aspx. Accessed June 27, 2017.

85. Centers for Medicare and Medicaid Services. *Hospice Determining Terminal Status-L33393.* 2015.

86.  Mitchell SL, Miller SC, Teno JM, Kiely DK, Davis RB, Shaffer ML. Prediction of 6-month survival of nursing home residents with advanced dementia using ADEPT vs hospice eligibility guidelines. *JAMA*. 2010;304(17):1929-1935.

87.  Sachs GA, Shega JW, Cox-Hayley D. Barriers to excellent end-of-life care for patients with dementia. *J Gen Intern Med*. 2004;19(10):1057-1063.

88.  Scherder E, Oosterman J, Swaab D, et al. Recent developments in pain in dementia. *BMJ*. 2005;330(7489):461-464.

89.  AGS Panel on Persistent Pain in Older Persons. The management of persistent pain in older persons. *J Am Geriatr Soc*. 2002;50(6 Suppl):S205-224.

90.  Taylor LJ, Herr K. Pain intensity assessment: a comparison of selected pain intensity scales for use in cognitively intact and cognitively impaired African American older adults. *Pain Manag Nurs*. 2003;4(2):87-95.

91.  Shega JW, Hougham GW, Stocking CB, Cox-Hayley D, Sachs GA. Pain in community-dwelling persons with dementia: frequency, intensity, and congruence between patient and caregiver report. *J Pain Symptom Manage*. 2004;28(6):585-592.

92.  Krulewitch H, London MR, Skakel VJ, Lundstedt GJ, Thomason H, Brummel-Smith K. Assessment of pain in cognitively impaired older adults: a comparison of pain assessment tools and their use by nonprofessional caregivers. *J Am Geriatr Soc*. 2000;48(12):1607-1611.

93.  Ferrell BA. Pain evaluation and management in the nursing home. *Ann Intern Med*. 1995;123(9):681-687.

94.  Won A, Lapane K, Gambassi G, Bernabei R, Mor V, Lipsitz LA. Correlates and management of nonmalignant pain in the nursing home. SAGE Study Group. Systematic Assessment of Geriatric drug use via Epidemiology. *J Am Geriatr Soc*. 1999;47(8):936-942.

95.  Hootman J, Bolen J, Helmick C, Langmaid G. Prevalence of doctor-diagnosed arthritis. *MMWR Morb Mortal Wkly Rep*. 2006;55(40):1089-1092. www.cdc.gov/mmwr/preview/mmwrhtml/mm5540a2.htm. Accessed June 29, 2017.

96.  Keenan AM, Tennant A, Fear J, Emery P, Conaghan PG. Impact of multiple joint problems on daily living tasks in people in the community over age fifty-five. *Arthritis Rheum*. 2006;55(5):757-764.

97.  Parmelee PA. Pain in cognitively impaired older persons. *Clin Geriatr Med*. 1996;12(3):473-487.

98.  Hurley AC, Volicer BJ, Hanrahan PA, Houde S, Volicer L. Assessment of discomfort in advanced Alzheimer patients. *Res Nurs Health*. 1992;15(5):369-377.

99.  Herr K, Bursch H, Ersek M, Miller LL, Swafford K. Use of pain-behavioral assessment tools in the nursing home: expert consensus recommendations for practice. *J Gerontol Nurs*. 2010;36(3):18-29.

100.  Feldt KS. The checklist of nonverbal pain indicators (CNPI). *Pain Manag Nurs*. 2000;1(1):13-21.

101.  Shega JW, Rudy T, Keefe FJ, Perri LC, Mengin OT, Weiner DK. Validity of pain behaviors in persons with mild to moderate cognitive impairment. *J Am Geriatr Soc*. 2008;56(9):1631-1637.

102.  Elliott AF, Horgas AL. Effects of an analgesic trial in reducing pain behaviors in community-dwelling older adults with dementia. *Nurs Res*. 2009;58(2):140-145.

103.  Manfredi PL, Breuer B, Wallenstein S, Stegmann M, Bottomley G, Libow L. Opioid treatment for agitation in patients with advanced dementia. *Int J Geriatr Psychiatry*. 2003;18(8):700-705.

104.  Ersek M, Cherrier MM, Overman SS, Irving GA. The cognitive effects of opioids. *Pain Manag Nurs*. 2004;5(2):75-93.

105.  Morrison RS, Magaziner J, Gilbert M, et al. Relationship between pain and opioid analgesics on the development of delirium following hip fracture. *J Gerontol A Biol Sci Med Sci*. 2003;58(1):76-81.

106.  Hollingworth P, Hamshere ML, Moskvina V, et al. Four components describe behavioral symptoms in 1,120 individuals with late-onset Alzheimer's disease. *J Am Geriatr Soc*. 2006;54(9):1348-1354.

107. Spalletta G, Musicco M, Padovani A, et al. Neuropsychiatric symptoms and syndromes in a large cohort of newly diagnosed, untreated patients with Alzheimer disease. *Am J Geriatr Psychiatry.* 2010;18(11):1026-1035.

108. Murman DL, Colenda CC. The economic impact of neuropsychiatric symptoms in Alzheimer's disease: can drugs ease the burden? *Pharmacoeconomics.* 2005;23(3):227-242.

109. McGivney SA, Mulvihill M, Taylor B. Validating the GDS depression screen in the nursing home. *J Am Geriatr Soc.* 1994;42(5):490-492.

110. Gerety MB, Williams JW, Jr., Mulrow CD, et al. Performance of case-finding tools for depression in the nursing home: influence of clinical and functional characteristics and selection of optimal threshold scores. *J Am Geriatr Soc.* 1994;42(10):1103-1109.

111. Alexopoulos GS, Abrams RC, Young RC, Shamoian CA. Cornell Scale for Depression in Dementia. *Biol Psychiatry.* 1988;23(3):271-284.

112. Sepehry AA, Lee PE, Hsiung GY, Beattie BL, Jacova C. Effect of selective serotonin reuptake inhibitors in Alzheimer's disease with comorbid depression: a meta-analysis of depression and cognitive outcomes. *Drugs Aging.* 2012;29(10):793-806.

113. Ballard CG, Patel A, Solis M, Lowe K, Wilcock G. A one-year follow-up study of depression in dementia sufferers. *Br J Psychiatry.* 1996;168(3):287-291.

114. Gruber-Baldini AL, Zimmerman S, Boustani M, Watson LC, Williams CS, Reed PS. Characteristics associated with depression in long-term care residents with dementia. *Gerontologist.* 2005;45(1):50-55.

115. Zubenko GS, Zubenko WN, McPherson S, et al. A collaborative study of the emergence and clinical features of the major depressive syndrome of Alzheimer's disease. *Am J Psychiatry.* 2003;160(5):857-866.

116. Karttunen K, Karppi P, Hiltunen A, et al. Neuropsychiatric symptoms and quality of life in patients with very mild and mild Alzheimer's disease. *Int J Geriatr Psychiatry.* 2011;26(5):473-482.

117. Ford AH, Almeida OP. Psychological treatment for depression and anxiety associated with dementia and mild cognitive impairment. *Br J Psychiatry.* 2015;207(4):286-287.

118. Forstl H, Burns A, Luthert P, Cairns N, Lantos P, Levy R. Clinical and neuropathological correlates of depression in Alzheimer's disease. *Psychol Med.* 1992;22(4):877-884.

119. Bains J, Birks JS, Dening TR. The efficacy of antidepressants in the treatment of depression in dementia. *Cochrane Database Syst Rev.* 2002(4):CD003944.

120. Modrego PJ. Depression in Alzheimer's disease. Pathophysiology, diagnosis, and treatment. *Journal of Alzheimer's disease : JAD.* 2010;21(4):1077-1087.

121. Katz IR, Simpson GM, Curlik SM, Parmelee PA, Muhly C. Pharmacologic treatment of major depression for elderly patients in residential care settings. *J Clin Psychiatry.* 1990;51 Suppl:41-47; discussion 48.

122. Galynker I, Ieronimo C, Miner C, Rosenblum J, Vilkas N, Rosenthal R. Methylphenidate treatment of negative symptoms in patients with dementia. *J Neuropsychiatry Clin Neurosci.* 1997;9(2):231-239.

123. Dolder CR, Davis LN, McKinsey J. Use of psychostimulants in patients with dementia. *Ann Pharmacother.* 2010;44(10):1624-1632.

124. Snowden M, Sato K, Roy-Byrne P. Assessment and treatment of nursing home residents with depression or behavioral symptoms associated with dementia: a review of the literature. *J Am Geriatr Soc.* 2003;51(9):1305-1317.

125. Hausner L, Damian M, Sartorius A, Frolich L. Efficacy and cognitive side effects of electroconvulsive therapy (ECT) in depressed elderly inpatients with coexisting mild cognitive impairment or dementia. *J Clin Psychiatry.* 2011;72(1):91-97.

126. Landes AM, Sperry SD, Strauss ME. Prevalence of apathy, dysphoria, and depression in relation to dementia severity in Alzheimer's disease. *J Neuropsychiatry Clin Neurosci.* 2005;17(3):342-349.

127. Landes AM, Sperry SD, Strauss ME, Geldmacher DS. Apathy in Alzheimer's disease. *J Am Geriatr Soc.* 2001;49(12):1700-1707.

128. Holmes C, Wilkinson D, Dean C, et al. The efficacy of donepezil in the treatment of neuropsychiatric symptoms in Alzheimer disease. *Neurology.* 2004;63(2):214-219.

129. Harrison F, Aerts L, Brodaty H. Apathy in Dementia: Systematic Review of Recent Evidence on Pharmacological Treatments. *Curr Psychiatry Rep.* 2016;18(11):103.

130. Peters KR, Rockwood K, Black SE, et al. Characterizing neuropsychiatric symptoms in subjects referred to dementia clinics. *Neurology.* 2006;66(4):523-528.

131. Craig D, Mirakhur A, Hart DJ, McIlroy SP, Passmore AP. A cross-sectional study of neuropsychiatric symptoms in 435 patients with Alzheimer's disease. *Am J Geriatr Psychiatry.* 2005;13(6):460-468.

132. Lyketsos CG, Lopez O, Jones B, Fitzpatrick AL, Breitner J, DeKosky S. Prevalence of neuropsychiatric symptoms in dementia and mild cognitive impairment: results from the cardiovascular health study. *JAMA.* 2002;288(12):1475-1483.

133. Del Ser T, McKeith I, Anand R, Cicin-Sain A, Ferrara R, Spiegel R. Dementia with lewy bodies: findings from an international multicentre study. *Int J Geriatr Psychiatry.* 2000;15(11):1034-1045.

134. Ropacki SA, Jeste DV. Epidemiology of and risk factors for psychosis of Alzheimer's disease: a review of 55 studies published from 1990 to 2003. *Am J Psychiatry.* 2005;162(11):2022-2030.

135. Paulsen JS, Salmon DP, Thal LJ, et al. Incidence of and risk factors for hallucinations and delusions in patients with probable AD. *Neurology.* 2000;54(10):1965-1971.

136. Schneider LS, Tariot PN, Dagerman KS, et al. Effectiveness of atypical antipsychotic drugs in patients with Alzheimer's disease. *N Engl J Med.* 2006;355(15):1525-1538.

137. Carson S, McDonagh MS, Peterson K. A systematic review of the efficacy and safety of atypical antipsychotics in patients with psychological and behavioral symptoms of dementia. *J Am Geriatr Soc.* 2006;54(2):354-361.

138. Schneider LS, Dagerman K, Insel PS. Efficacy and adverse effects of atypical antipsychotics for dementia: meta-analysis of randomized, placebo-controlled trials. *Am J Geriatr Psychiatry.* 2006;14(3):191-210.

139. Agar MR, Lawlor PG, Quinn S, et al. Efficacy of Oral Risperidone, Haloperidol, or Placebo for Symptoms of Delirium Among Patients in Palliative Care: A Randomized Clinical Trial. *JAMA Intern Med.* 2017;177(1):34-42.

140. Rosenheck RA, Leslie DL, Sindelar JL, et al. Cost-benefit analysis of second-generation antipsychotics and placebo in a randomized trial of the treatment of psychosis and aggression in Alzheimer disease. *Arch Gen Psychiatry.* 2007;64(11):1259-1268.

141. Jeste DV, Blazer D, Casey D, et al. ACNP White Paper: update on use of antipsychotic drugs in elderly persons with dementia. *Neuropsychopharmacology.* 2008;33(5):957-970.

142. Schneider LS, Dagerman KS, Insel P. Risk of death with atypical antipsychotic drug treatment for dementia: meta-analysis of randomized placebo-controlled trials. *JAMA.* 2005;294(15):1934-1943.

143. Cohen-Mansfield J, Thein K, Marx MS. Predictors of the impact of nonpharmacologic interventions for agitation in nursing home residents with advanced dementia. *J Clin Psychiatry.* 2014;75(7):e666-671.

144. Devanand DP, Mintzer J, Schultz SK, et al. Relapse risk after discontinuation of risperidone in Alzheimer's disease. *N Engl J Med.* 2012;367(16):1497-1507.

145. Ballard CG, Gauthier S, Cummings JL, et al. Management of agitation and aggression associated with Alzheimer disease. *Nat Rev Neurol.* 2009;5(5):245-255.

146. Jeste DV, Meeks TW, Kim DS, Zubenko GS. Research agenda for DSM-V: diagnostic categories and criteria for neuropsychiatric syndromes in dementia. *J Geriatr Psychiatry Neurol.* 2006;19(3):160-171.

147. Stern TA, Celano CM, Gross AF, et al. The assessment and management of agitation and delirium in the general hospital. *Prim Care Companion J Clin Psychiatry*. 2010;12(1):PCC.09r00938.

148. Cohen-Mansfield J, Marx MS, Werner P. Agitation in elderly persons: an integrative report of findings in a nursing home. *Int Psychogeriatr*. 1992;4 Suppl 2:221-240.

149. Hope T, Keene J, Fairburn C, McShane R, Jacoby R. Behaviour changes in dementia: are there behavioural syndromes? *Int J Geriatr Psychiatry*. 1997;12(11):1074-1078.

150. Hamel M, Gold DP, Andres D, et al. Predictors and consequences of aggressive behavior by community-based dementia patients. *Gerontologist*. 1990;30(2):206-211.

151. Deutsch LH, Bylsma FW, Rovner BW, Steele C, Folstein MF. Psychosis and physical aggression in probable Alzheimer's disease. *Am J Psychiatry*. 1991;148(9):1159-1163.

152. McMinn B, Draper B. Vocally disruptive behaviour in dementia: development of an evidence based practice guideline. *Aging Ment Health*. 2005;9(1):16-24.

153. Ayalon L, Gum AM, Feliciano L, Arean PA. Effectiveness of nonpharmacological interventions for the management of neuropsychiatric symptoms in patients with dementia: a systematic review. *Arch Intern Med*. 2006;166(20):2182-2188.

154. Gitlin LN, Winter L, Dennis MP, Hodgson N, Hauck WW. Targeting and managing behavioral symptoms in individuals with dementia: a randomized trial of a nonpharmacological intervention. *J Am Geriatr Soc*. 2010;58(8):1465-1474.

155. Cohen-Mansfield J, Marx MS, Dakheel-Ali M, Regier NG, Thein K, Freedman L. Can agitated behavior of nursing home residents with dementia be prevented with the use of standardized stimuli? *J Am Geriatr Soc*. 2010;58(8):1459-1464.

156. Martinon-Torres G, Fioravanti M, Grimley EJ. Trazodone for agitation in dementia. *Cochrane Database Syst Rev*. 2004(4):CD004990.

157. Sultzer DL, Gray KF, Gunay I, Berisford MA, Mahler ME. A double-blind comparison of trazodone and haloperidol for treatment of agitation in patients with dementia. *Am J Geriatr Psychiatry*. 1997;5(1):60-69.

158. Pollock BG, Mulsant BH, Rosen J, et al. Comparison of citalopram, perphenazine, and placebo for the acute treatment of psychosis and behavioral disturbances in hospitalized, demented patients. *Am J Psychiatry*. 2002;159(3):460-465.

159. Gauthier S, Wirth Y, Mobius HJ. Effects of memantine on behavioural symptoms in Alzheimer's disease patients: an analysis of the Neuropsychiatric Inventory (NPI) data of two randomised, controlled studies. *Int J Geriatr Psychiatry*. 2005;20(5):459-464.

160. Kirven LE, Montero EF. Comparison of thioridazine and diazepam in the control of nonpsychotic symptoms associated with senility: double-blind study. *J Am Geriatr Soc*. 1973;21(12):546-551.

161. Lonergan ET, Cameron M, Luxenberg J. Valproic acid for agitation in dementia. *Cochrane Database Syst Rev*. 2004(2):CD003945.

162. Tariot PN, Erb R, Podgorski CA, et al. Efficacy and tolerability of carbamazepine for agitation and aggression in dementia. *Am J Psychiatry*. 1998;155(1):54-61.

163. Miller LJ. Gabapentin for treatment of behavioral and psychological symptoms of dementia. *Ann Pharmacother*. 2001;35(4):427-431.

164. van den Elsen GA, Ahmed AI, Verkes RJ, et al. Tetrahydrocannabinol for neuropsychiatric symptoms in dementia: A randomized controlled trial. *Neurology*. 2015;84(23):2338-2346.

165. Cummings JL, Lyketsos CG, Peskind ER, et al. Effect of Dextromethorphan-Quinidine on Agitation in Patients With Alzheimer Disease Dementia: A Randomized Clinical Trial. *JAMA*. 2015;314(12):1242-1254.

166. Ganguli M, Rodriguez EG. Reporting of dementia on death certificates: a community study. *J Am Geriatr Soc*. 1999;47(7):842-849.

167. Mitchell SL, Kiely DK, Hamel MB. Dying with advanced dementia in the nursing home. *Arch Intern Med.* 2004;164(3):321-326.

168. Mitchell SL, Morris JN, Park PS, Fries BE. Terminal care for persons with advanced dementia in the nursing home and home care settings. *J Palliat Med.* 2004;7(6):808-816.

169. Baer WM, Hanson LC. Families' perception of the added value of hospice in the nursing home. *J Am Geriatr Soc.* 2000;48(8):879-882.

170. Munn JC, Hanson LC, Zimmerman S, Sloane PD, Mitchell CM. Is hospice associated with improved end-of-life care in nursing homes and assisted living facilities? *J Am Geriatr Soc.* 2006;54(3):490-495.

171. Miller SC, Mor V, Teno J. Hospice enrollment and pain assessment and management in nursing homes. *J Pain Symptom Manage.* 2003;26(3):791-799.

172. Shega JW, Hougham GW, Stocking CB, Cox-Hayley D, Sachs GA. Management of noncancer pain in community-dwelling persons with dementia. *J Am Geriatr Soc.* 2006;54(12):1892-1897.

173. Hanson LC, Zimmerman S, Song MK, et al. Effect of the Goals of Care Intervention for Advanced Dementia: A Randomized Clinical Trial. *JAMA Int Med.* 2017;177(1):24-31.

174. Volicer L, Seltzer B, Rheaume Y, et al. Eating difficulties in patients with probable dementia of the Alzheimer type. *J Geriatr Psychiatry Neurol.* 1989;2(4):188-195.

175. Volicer L, Rheaume Y, Cyr D. Treatment of depression in advanced Alzheimer's disease using sertraline. *J Geriatr Psychiatry Neurol.* 1994;7(4):227-229.

176. Bosley BN, Weiner DK, Rudy TE, Granieri E. Is chronic nonmalignant pain associated with decreased appetite in older adults? Preliminary evidence. *J Am Geriatr Soc.* 2004;52(2):247-251.

177. Callahan CM, Haag KM, Weinberger M, et al. Outcomes of percutaneous endoscopic gastrostomy among older adults in a community setting. *J Am Geriatr Soc.* 2000;48(9):1048-1054.

178. Finucane TE, Christmas C, Travis K. Tube feeding in patients with advanced dementia: a review of the evidence. *JAMA.* 1999;282(14):1365-1370.

179. Gillick MR. Rethinking the role of tube feeding in patients with advanced dementia. *N Engl J Med.* 2000;342(3):206-210.

180. Mitchell SL, Mor V, Gozalo PL, Servadio JL, Teno JM. Tube Feeding in US Nursing Home Residents With Advanced Dementia, 2000-2014. *JAMA.* 2016;316(7):769-770.

181. Shega JW, Hougham GW, Stocking CB, Cox-Hayley D, Sachs GA. Barriers to limiting the practice of feeding tube placement in advanced dementia. *J Palliat Med.* 2003;6(6):885-893.

182. Candy B, Sampson EL, Jones L. Enteral tube feeding in older people with advanced dementia: findings from a Cochrane systematic review. *Int J Palliat Nurs.* 2009;15(8):396-404.

183. Meier DE, Ahronheim JC, Morris J, Baskin-Lyons S, Morrison RS. High short-term mortality in hospitalized patients with advanced dementia: lack of benefit of tube feeding. *Arch Intern Med.* 2001;161(4):594-599.

184. Kuo S, Rhodes RL, Mitchell SL, Mor V, Teno JM. Natural history of feeding-tube use in nursing home residents with advanced dementia. *J Am Med Dir Assoc.* 2009;10(4):264-270.

185. Finucane TE, Bynum JP. Use of tube feeding to prevent aspiration pneumonia. *Lancet.* 1996;348(9039):1421-1424.

186. American Geriatrics Society feeding tubes in advanced dementia position statement. *J Am Geriatr Soc.* 2014;62(8):1590-1593.

187. Volandes AE, Paasche-Orlow MK, Barry MJ, et al. Video decision support tool for advance care planning in dementia: randomised controlled trial. *BMJ.* 2009;338:b2159.

188. Teno JM, Gozalo P, Mitchell SL, Tyler D, Mor V. Survival after multiple hospitalizations for infections and dehydration in nursing home residents with advanced cognitive impairment. *JAMA.* 2013;310(3):319-320.

189. Dufour AB, Shaffer ML, D'Agata EM, Habtemariam D, Mitchell SL. Survival after suspected urinary tract infection in individuals with advanced dementia. *J Am Geriatr Soc.* 2015;63(12):2472-2477.

190. Morrison RS, Ahronheim JC, Morrison GR, et al. Pain and discomfort associated with common hospital procedures and experiences. *J Pain Symptom Manage.* 1998;15(2):91-101.

191. van der Steen JT, Kruse RL, Ooms ME, et al. Treatment of nursing home residents with dementia and lower respiratory tract infection in the United States and The Netherlands: an ocean apart. *J Am Geriatr Soc.* 2004;52(5):691-699.

192. Fabiszewski KJ, Volicer B, Volicer L. Effect of antibiotic treatment on outcome of fevers in institutionalized Alzheimer patients. *JAMA.* 1990;263(23):3168-3172.

193. Givens JL, Jones RN, Shaffer ML, Kiely DK, Mitchell SL. Survival and comfort after treatment of pneumonia in advanced dementia. *Arch Intern Med.* 2010;170(13):1102-1107.

194. Morrison RS, Siu AL. A comparison of pain and its treatment in advanced dementia and cognitively intact patients with hip fracture. *J Pain Symptom Manage.* 2000;19(4):240-248.

195. Feldt KS, Ryden MB, Miles S. Treatment of pain in cognitively impaired compared with cognitively intact older patients with hip-fracture. *J Am Geriatr Soc.* 1998;46(9):1079-1085.

196. Alexander GC, Sayla MA, Holmes HM, Sachs GA. Prioritizing and stopping prescription medicines. *CMAJ.* 2006;174(8):1083-1084.

197. Holmes HM, Hayley DC, Alexander GC, Sachs GA. Reconsidering medication appropriateness for patients late in life. *Arch Intern Med.* 2006;166(6):605-609.

198. Scott IA, Hilmer SN, Reeve E, et al. Reducing inappropriate polypharmacy: the process of deprescribing. *JAMA internal medicine.* 2015;175(5):827-834.

199. Volicer L, Rheaume Y, Brown J, Fabiszewski K, Brady R. Hospice approach to the treatment of patients with advanced dementia of the Alzheimer type. *JAMA.* 1986;256(16):2210-2213.

200. Shega JW, Hougham GW, Stocking CB, Cox-Hayley D, Sachs GA. Patients dying with dementia: experience at the end of life and impact of hospice care. *J Pain Symptom Manage.* 2008;35(5):499-507.

201. Schulz R, Mendelsohn AB, Haley WE, et al. End-of-life care and the effects of bereavement on family caregivers of persons with dementia. *N Engl J Med.* 2003;349(20):1936-1942.

202. Brown MA, Sampson EL, Jones L, Barron AM. Prognostic indicators of 6-month mortality in elderly people with advanced dementia: a systematic review. *Palliat Med.* 2013;27(5):389-400.

203. Miller SC, Mor V, Wu N, Gozalo P, Lapane K. Does receipt of hospice care in nursing homes improve the management of pain at the end of life? *J Am Geriatr Soc.* 2002;50(3):507-515.

204. Kiely DK, Givens JL, Shaffer ML, Teno JM, Mitchell SL. Hospice use and outcomes in nursing home residents with advanced dementia. *J Am Geriatr Soc.* 2010;58(12):2284-2291.

205. Ory MG, Hoffman RR, 3rd, Yee JL, Tennstedt S, Schulz R. Prevalence and impact of caregiving: a detailed comparison between dementia and nondementia caregivers. *Gerontologist.* 1999;39(2):177-185.

206. Schulz R, Newsom J, Mittelmark M, Burton L, Hirsch C, Jackson S. Health effects of caregiving: the caregiver health effects study: an ancillary study of the Cardiovascular Health Study. *Ann Behav Med.* 1997;19(2):110-116.

207. Mahoney R, Regan C, Katona C, Livingston G. Anxiety and depression in family caregivers of people with Alzheimer disease: the LASER-AD study. *Am J Geriatr Psychiatry.* 2005;13(9):795-801.

208. Schulz R, Beach SR. Caregiving as a risk factor for mortality: the Caregiver Health Effects Study. *JAMA.* 1999;282(23):2215-2219.

209. Yee JL, Schulz R. Gender differences in psychiatric morbidity among family caregivers: a review and analysis. *Gerontologist.* 2000;40(2):147-164.

210. Irwin SA, Mausbach BT, Koo D, et al. Association between hospice care and psychological outcomes in Alzheimer's spousal caregivers. *J Palliat Med.* 2013;16(11):1450-1454.

211. Yaffe K, Fox P, Newcomer R, et al. Patient and caregiver characteristics and nursing home placement in patients with dementia. *JAMA.* 2002;287(16):2090-2097.

212. Schulz R, Belle SH, Czaja SJ, McGinnis KA, Stevens A, Zhang S. Long-term care placement of dementia patients and caregiver health and well-being. *JAMA.* 2004;292(8):961-967.

213. Gitlin LN, Belle SH, Burgio LD, et al. Effect of multicomponent interventions on caregiver burden and depression: the REACH multisite initiative at 6-month follow-up. *Psychol Aging.* 2003;18(3):361-374.

214. Rabinowitz YG, Mausbach BT, Coon DW, Depp C, Thompson LW, Gallagher-Thompson D. The moderating effect of self-efficacy on intervention response in women family caregivers of older adults with dementia. *Am J Geriatr Psychiatry.* 2006;14(8):642-649.

215. Belle SH, Burgio L, Burns R, et al. Enhancing the quality of life of dementia caregivers from different ethnic or racial groups: a randomized, controlled trial. *Ann Intern Med.* 2006;145(10):727-738.

216. Elliott AF, Burgio LD, Decoster J. Enhancing caregiver health: findings from the resources for enhancing Alzheimer's caregiver health II intervention. *J Am Geriatr Soc.* 2010;58(1):30-37.

217. Sorensen S, Pinquart M, Duberstein P. How effective are interventions with caregivers? An updated meta-analysis. *Gerontologist.* 2002;42(3):356-372.

218. Blom MM, Zarit SH, Groot Zwaaftink RB, Cuijpers P, Pot AM. Effectiveness of an Internet intervention for family caregivers of people with dementia: results of a randomized controlled trial. *PLoS One.* 2015;10(2):e0116622.

219. Schulz R, Boerner K, Shear K, Zhang S, Gitlin LN. Predictors of complicated grief among dementia caregivers: a prospective study of bereavement. *Am J Geriatr Psychiatry.* 2006;14(8):650-658.

# Neurological Conditions

## Palliative Neurology: Introduction, Definitions, and Diagnostic Criteria

In the field of neurology, there are many diseases that are chronic, progressive, life-limiting, and very disabling, which is where the bridge between palliative care and neurology exist. Although palliative care emerged in the treatment of patients with underlying malignancy and then expanded to chronic illness such as heart failure, chronic obstructive pulmonary disease, and end-stage renal disease, a later but emerging interest is how to apply palliative care principles to the care of patients with underlying neurological conditions.[1-9] Conditions such as stroke, epilepsy, seizures, movement disorders (Parkinson's disease [PD]), demyelinating diseases (multiple sclerosis [MS]), neuromuscular disorders (amyotrophic lateral sclerosis [ALS]), neuromuscular junction disorders (myasthenia gravis), myopathy disorders (Duchenne muscular dystrophy), and nervous system malignancies (glioblastoma) can result in physical, emotional, and existential symptoms that can be particularly challenging to manage.[2,9-11]

It is especially difficult not just for the patients but also for their loved ones as progressive neurological conditions lead to loss of function, communication difficulties, personality and memory changes, and ultimately shortened prognosis. The care of patients with serious and progressive neurological conditions presents numerous opportunities to integrate palliative care from diagnosis to end of life. Palliative care providers can play an active role by improving overall quality of life (QOL) with a focus on physical, psychological, social, and spiritual issues of these patients, along with improving communication, advance care planning, and, eventually, end-of-life care. This is especially true for critically ill patients with neurological disease or patients who have a critical illness involving the neuromuscular system, spinal cord, or brain.[12] These illnesses often occur after a catastrophic sudden event, with many patients never regaining functional independence, resulting in sustained permanent disabilities. It's also important that clinicians address the caregiver's well-being because they ultimately play a vital role in the health of patients with underlying neurological conditions.

Unfortunately, even though these diseases can be very disabling with high symptom burden, many neurologists lack the education and expertise in palliative care, and fewer than 2% of palliative care clinicians are neurologists, which has contributed to the underutilization of palliative care for patients with underlying neurological conditions.[2,4,13] The heterogeneity of progression, limited efficacy of symptomatic treatment, lack of reliable prognostic markers, and the high prevalence of communication and cognitive impairments also have contributed to the underutilization of palliative care. Thus, an interdisciplinary team approach is essential for this care population, along with the expansion of training in primary palliative care.[13] The American Academy of Neurology Ethics and Humanities Subcommittee stated in 1996 that "Many patients with neurologic disease die after long illnesses during which a neurologist acts as the principal or consulting physician. Therefore, it is imperative that neurologists understand, and learn to apply, the principles of palliative medicine."[1,14] Similarly, the Accreditation Council for Graduate Medical Education requires neurology residents to receive instruction in palliative and end-of-life care.[15] It is important to improve primary and specialist level palliative care for patients with underlying neurological conditions. [16,17]

## *Definitions and Diagnostic Criteria*
### Stroke

Stroke is the most common life-threatening neurological disease. It is the fifth leading cause of death in the United Sates (after heart disease, cancer, chronic respiratory disease, and accidents), affecting approximately 6.3 million adults.[18-20] A stroke is the rapid loss of neurologic function in a particular vascular territory, with symptoms lasting greater than 24 hours. Strokes either result from ischemic or hemorrhagic causes.[21,22] Ischemic strokes are classified into categories according to their pathophysiologic type of lesion and mechanism of ischemic brain injury, such as large artery atherosclerotic infarct, embolic, small vessel, undetermined cause (cryptogenic), or other determined causes (eg, dissection).[20,23]

Hemorrhagic strokes are classified according to their location, pathophysiologic type, and cause. Hemorrhage can occur in the ventricular system (intraventricular hemorrhage), subarachnoid space (subarachnoid hemorrhage), or brain parenchyma (intracerebral hemorrhage). Further classification occurs for intracerebral hemorrhages as either primary or secondary types. The most common primary causes are hypertension, medications (especially antiplatelet, anticoagulant, and thrombolytic), and cerebral amyloid angiopathy.[12,20,23] Some secondary causes are vasculitis, aneurysms, neoplasms, hemorrhagic transformation, malformations, and cerebral venous sinus thrombosis. Neuroimaging helps to differentiate ischemic stroke from hemorrhagic stroke. There are multiple stroke diagnostic scales available to aid in identification of an acute stroke including the Face Arm Speech Test (FAST), the Cincinnati Prehospital Stroke Scale (CPSS), the Los Angeles Prehospital Stroke Screen (LAPSS), and the Recognition of Stroke in the Emergency Room (ROSIER).[24]

### Movement Disorders

Movement disorders are a broad class of conditions generally classified and differentiated on the basis of clinical factors. The major categories of abnormal movements include tremor, dystonia, chorea, ataxia, myoclonus, and parkinsonism.[20,25] A tremor is a rhythmic oscillation of a body part which is differentiated on the basis of frequency, location, and presence at rest, with movement or sustained posture.[26] Dystonia is characterized by sustained or intermittent contractions of the muscle, causing abnormal, often repetitive movements, postures, or both. It can involve virtually any body part.[27] Chorea is brief, irregular, nonrhythmic movements involving extremities, head, trunk, or face.[20,28] Ataxia is an impairment of initiation and coordination of movements that can involve gait, speech, and extremities.[29] Myoclonus is characterized by brief, lightning-like involuntary jerking caused by muscular contractions or inhibitions.[30] Parkinsonism is a set of clinical features that include rigidity, resting tremor, bradykinesia, and postural instability. The major types of movement disorders and key features can be seen in **Table 17**.

Key diagnostic criteria for movement disorders are based on a clinician's ability to recognize the characteristic signs and associated symptoms. Huntington's disease (HD) stands out as one of the most devastating illnesses, not only because of its incurable neurodegenerative progression that occurs over many years but also its impact on families. HD is the most common hereditary neurodegenerative disorder.[32] Symptoms often start when patients are in their 30s and 40s, and there is progression over time in cognitive, psychiatric, and motor changes (especially chorea) with mean duration of 15 to 20 years from the time of onset to death.[37] Almost one-third of patients will require treatment in a long-term-care facility.[38] Since HD is autosomal dominant, children have a 50% chance of developing the disease themselves, and studies find that up to 40% of children report HD as having major, negative consequences on their families.[38] The other devastating feature of HD is that there are no curative or disease-modifying treatments currently available, making supportive care the only option.

This section will focus on Parkinson's disease, or PD (see **Table 18** for diagnostic criteria).[39] Also, the DaTscan, which is a dopamine transporter single photon emission computerized tomography (SPECT) imaging technique, can be a useful tool to help diagnose PD, especially in patients with unclear symptoms.[40]

### Demyelinating Disorders

Demyelinating disorders are a group of immune mediated conditions affecting the myelin of the central nervous system (CNS). The peripheral nervous system is spared. MS is the most common disease in this category, second to trauma as a major cause of neurologic disability in early- to middle-age adults.[20,42,43] The other major diseases in this category are neuromyelitis optica, acute disseminated encephalomyelitis, and transverse myelitis. MS is a chronic condition characterized by recurrent episodes of demyelination in the CNS. The CNS lesions of MS typically develop at different times and in different locations. Patients will also have inflammation, gliosis, and neuronal loss. The clinical deficits that occur will depend on the location of the inflammation and demyelination, and the course can be relapsing-remitting or progressive. The McDonald Criteria is used to diagnosis MS.[43] It has identified two major criteria: (a) the presence of two or more attacks and (b) objective evidence of two or more neurological lesions. If these two criteria are not met, additional evidence is needed. Magnetic resonance imaging (MRI) is the preferred test to support the clinical diagnosis of MS.[44]

### Neuromuscular Disorders

Neuromuscular disorders encompass several different neurological conditions that impair the peripheral nervous system. The main categories of neuromuscular disorders consist of peripheral neuropathies (Guillain-Barre syndrome), motor neuron disorders (ALS), neuromuscular junction disorders (myasthenia gravis) and myopathies (Duchenne muscular dystrophy).

## Table 17. Major Movement Disorders

| Disorder | Key Features |
|---|---|
| PD | Postural instability, asymmetric resting tremor, bradykinesia, and rigidity (In presence of early falls, early dementia, early autonomic dysfunction, ataxia, rapid progression, and/or poor response to levodopa, think alternative diagnosis.)[25] |
| Drug-induced parkinsonism | Bilateral postural tremor, bradykinesia, and rigidity[25] |
| Dementia with Lewy body | Cognitive fluctuations, prior onset of parkinsonism features, visual hallucinations, REM sleep disorder, and severe neuroleptic sensitivity[31] |
| Huntington's disease | Hereditary (autosomal dominant), severe motor impairment (especially chorea), cognitive decline, and psychiatric symptoms[32] |
| Multiple system atrophy | Autonomic dysfunction (especially genitourinary symptoms), rapid progression of parkinsonism features with poor response to levodopa, cerebellar syndrome (gait ataxia, dysarthria, limb ataxia, or cerebellar oculomotor dysfunction)<br><br>Atrophy on MRI in putamen, middle cerebellar peduncle, pons, or cerebellum[16] |
| Progressive supranuclear palsy | Supranuclear ophthalmoparesis or plegia, postural instability, and falls<br><br>Dysarthria, dysphagia, pseudobulbar palsy, rigidity, frontal cognitive abnormalities, and sleep disturbances are additional common clinical features.[33,34] |
| Restless leg syndrome | Unpleasant or uncomfortable sensation in the legs that occurs at rest, especially in the evening, causing irresistible urge to move one's legs[35] |
| Periodic limb movements | Rhythmic twitches of the legs that occur during sleep[36] |

*MRI, manetic resonance imaging; PD, Parkinson's disease; REM, rapid eye movement*

## Table 18. Diagnostic Criteria for Parkinson's Disease[39]

First the diagnosis of parkinsonism must be confirmed using the Movement Disorder Society (MDS) Unified Parkinson's Disease Rating Scale.[41] Then diagnosis of clinically established PD requires

1. absence of absolute exclusion criteria
2. at least two supportive criteria
3. no red flags (at least no more than two; presence of red flags must be counterbalanced by supportive criteria)

**Supportive Criteria**

1. Clear and dramatic beneficial response to dopaminergic therapy
2. Presence of levodopa-induced dyskinesia
3. Resting tremor of a limb
4. The presence of either olfactory loss or cardiac sympathetic denervation on MIBG scintigraphy

**Absolute Exclusion Criteria (presence of any of these rules out PD)**

- Unequivocal cerebellar abnormalities (eg, cerebellar gait, limb ataxia, cerebellar oculomotor abnormalities)
- Diagnosis of behavioral variant of frontotemporal dementia or primary progressive aphasia within the first 5 years of disease
- Treatment with a dopamine receptor blocker or dopamine depleting agent in dose and time consistent with drug-induced parkinsonism
- Unequivocal cortical sensory loss (ie, graphesthesia), clear limb ideomotor apraxia, or progressive aphasia

- Documentation of an alternative condition known to cause parkinsonism
- Downward vertical supranuclear gaze palsy or downward vertical saccades
- Parkinsonian features restricted to the lower limbs for more than 3 years
- Absence of observable response to high dose levodopa
- Normal functional neuroimaging of the presynaptic dopaminergic system

*Continued on page 110*

## Table 18. Diagnostic Criteria for Parkinson's Disease[39] *(continued)*

**Red Flags**

- Rapid progression of gait impairment requiring wheelchair within 5 years of onset
- Early bulbar dysfunction: severe dystonia, dysarthria, severe dysphagia within first 5 years
- Severe autonomic failure in the first 5 years
- Disproportionate anterocollis (dystonic) or contractures on hands or feet within first 10 years
- Otherwise unexplained pyramidal tract signs

- Complete absence of progression motor symptoms/signs over 5 years, unless stability related to treatment
- Inspiratory respiratory dysfunction
- Recurrent (> 1/year) falls because of impaired balance within 3 years of onset
- Absence of any of the common non-motor features despite 5 years of disease (sleep dysfunction, autonomic dysfunction, hyposmia, or psychiatric dysfunction)
- Bilateral symmetric parkinsonism

*MIBG, iodine-123-meta-iodobenzylguanidine*
*Adapted from MDS clinical diagnostic criteria for Parkinson's disease, by Postuma RB, Berg D, Stern M, et al., Mov Disord, 2015;30(12):1591-1601. © John Wiley and Sons, Inc. Adapted with permission.*

Patients experience a range of symptoms depending on the etiology, including but not limited to muscle weakness, loss of muscle mass, double vision, and difficulty breathing. For this section, we will focus on ALS, also known by the eponym Lou Gehrig's disease. ALS is diagnosed using the revised El Escorial World Federation of Neurology criteria, also known as the Airlie House criteria.[45,46] For a definitive diagnosis, the patient must have lower motor neuron signs (weakness, muscular atrophy, reduced reflexes) plus upper motor neuron signs (spasticity, increased reflexes) in at least three regions. CNS pathology seen in ALS includes frontal cortical atrophy, degeneration of both the corticospinal and spinocerebellar tracts, a reduction in large cervical and lumbar motor neurons, and cranial nerve nuclei degeneration.

## Key Points

One of the major challenges presented by diseases such as PD and ALS is that the diagnosis is mostly clinical. Unlike cancer, there is no demonstrable pathology, and often the diagnosis for neurologic conditions is not found for years, leading to significant psychosocial distress for the patients and their loved ones. **Table 19** provides a comparison of the more common neurologic conditions.

# Table 19. Comparison of Common Neurological Conditions

| Disease | Signs/Symptoms | Pathophysiology | Diagnosis |
|---------|----------------|-----------------|-----------|
| Stroke | Rapid onset of focal (or global, as in subarachnoid hemorrhage) cerebral deficit, lasting more than 24 hours, with no apparent cause other than a vascular one | Often underlying cardiac or blood vessel disease.<br><br>Ischemic strokes are often secondary to either a thrombus, emboli, or global ischemia (hypotension). Some other causes include vasospasm, dissection, or arteritis.<br><br>Hemorrhagic strokes can occur from leakage from intracerebral arteries chronic hypertension, bleeding diatheses, medications (anticoagulants, cocaine), cerebral amyloidosis, increased ICP, aneurysm, or AVMs. | CT and/or MRI |
| PD | Postural instability, asymmetric resting tremor, bradykinesia and rigidity<br><br>Nonmotor symptoms include hyposmia, rapid eye movements, sleep behavior disorders, personality changes, pain, paresthesia, and depression.<br><br>Late onset motor symptoms (postural instability, falls, freezing of gait, speech and swallowing difficulties) along with urinary disturbances, orthostatic hypotension, and neuropsychiatric disturbances (dementia, hallucination, delirium) often occur later in the disease course. | Progressive loss of dopamine containing neurons of the pars compacta of the substantia nigra, which causes denervation of the nigrostriatal tract and significant reduction of dopamine at the striatal level.<br><br>The consequence of this denervation process is an imbalance in the striatopallidal and pallidothalamic output pathways, which is responsible for the major motor deficit.<br><br>The presence of Lewy bodies (cytoplasmic proteinaceous inclusion) in surviving dopaminergic neurons is the pathological hallmark of PD. | MDS-Unified PD Rating Scale[41]<br><br>DaTscan also can help with diagnosis. |

*Continued on page 112*

## Table 19. Comparison of Common Neurological Conditions *(continued)*

| Disease | Signs/Symptoms | Pathophysiology | Diagnosis |
|---|---|---|---|
| MS | Virtually any CNS symptom can occur in MS.<br><br>Course is relapsing-remitting or progressive.<br><br>Ascending sensory symptoms (paresthesia of limbs/face), optic neuritis (monocular loss of vision associated with optic pain and impaired color vision), oculomotor dysfunction (diplopia, oscillopsia, internuclear ophthalmoplegia), motor weakness, bladder/bowel dysfunction, imbalance, facial pain<br><br>A characteristic symptom includes Lhermitte Sign (limb or spinal paresthesia elicited by neck flexion), along with heat and exercise sensitivity. | Autoimmune<br><br>Demyelinating lesions (plaques) involving the white matter episodically occurring in the brain, spinal cord and/or optic nerve<br><br>Pathological hallmark of MS plaques are inflammation and demyelination with relative sparing of nerve axons.<br><br>Often see complement activation, immunoglobulin deposition, loss of oligodendrocytes, and/or apoptosis | McDonald Criteria[43]<br><br>Major criteria: presence of two or more attacks with objective evidence of two or more neurological lesions.<br><br>MRI is the preferred test to support the clinical diagnosis of MS. |
| ALS | Presence of lower motor neuron signs (weakness, muscular atrophy, and fasciculations), gait disorders (steppage or waddling), reduced reflexes plus upper motor neuron signs (spasticity, increased reflexes, slowed rapid alternating movements, gait disorders [spastic], clonus) | There are familial and sporadic types of ALS.<br><br>Characterized by motor neuron degeneration, gliosis, and axonal loss in corticospinal tract<br><br>Intracellular inclusions in degenerating neurons and glia are frequent neuropathological findings of ALS. | Revised El Escorial World Federation of Neurology criteria, also known as the Airlie House criteria[45,46] |

*ALS, amyotrophic lateral sclerosis; AVM, arteriovenous malformation; CNS, central nervous system; CT, computed tomography; ICP, intracranial pressure; MRI, magnetic resonance imaging; MS, multiple sclerosis; PD, Parkinson's disease*

## Susan

Susan is a 72-year-old woman with a medical history of high blood pressure, diabetes, osteoarthritis, and dyslipidemia. She also has a history of smoking (20 packs per year) and is a retired school teacher. She lives with her husband and is independent in all her ADLs and IADLs. Susan suddenly developed acute onset of difficulty talking and right-sided weakness. The family members who witnessed the onset said that the symptoms progressed over a few minutes and that they were accompanied by nausea, vomiting, and headache. Susan was brought to the emergency department 1 hour after the onset. Her only medications at home are acetaminophen 1,000 mg orally twice a day, and lisinopril. During physical exam, she is very difficult to arouse and continues to vomit repeatedly. Her blood pressure is elevated at 210/105, pulse is 104/min, and respiration rate is 20. There is no nuchal rigidity, no carotid bruits, and no jugular venous distention. She has global aphasia and right hemiplegia. The rest of the exam is unremarkable.

 Based on your clinical evaluation, what diagnoses should be considered at this time?

This patient most likely has had intracerebral hemorrhage. The classic triad is sudden onset of a focal neurologic deficit with subsequent symptomatic progression over minutes to hours. The presence of headache, vomiting, hypertension, and impaired level of consciousness helps distinguish it from an ischemic stroke. Intracerebral hemorrhages account for about 11% of stroke deaths. One-month mortality rate is as high as 35% to 52%. The next step would be to order a computed tomography (CT) and MRI/magnetic resonance angiography (MRA) of the brain. This will help provide diagnostics and prognostic information.

A severe ischemic stroke generally does not progress or worsen as rapidly as it did in this patient. Transient ischemic attacks (TIAs) are brief episodes of focal neurologic dysfunction without progression and last less than 30 minutes. Meningitis is very unlikely given this presentation as well as the absence of fever and nuchal rigidity. MS also is unlikely given this presentation and age of this patient. Patients with MS can present with acute transverse myelitis, but the symptoms typically are rapid onset of bilateral weakness, sensory alternations, and bowel or bladder dysfunction below the level of the lesion.

 What factors are important in estimating Susan's mortality rate after this acute intracerebral hemorrhage?

The volume of intracranial hemorrhage and level of consciousness are the two most important predictors of outcomes in this setting. In addition, age, location of hemorrhage, and presence of an intraventricular hemorrhage are also important. The intracerebral hemorrhage (ICH) scores can also be used to estimate mortality (0 = best, 6 = worst; each point equates to 13% 30-day mortality rate)[47]:

| | |
|---|---|
| Glasgow Coma Scale (GCS) | 3-4 (2 points), 5-12 (1 point), 13-15 (0 points) |
| Age | ≥ 80 years (1 point) |
| ICH Volume ≥ 30 mL | 1 point |
| Intraventricular hemorrhage | 1 point |
| Infratentorial origin of hemorrhage | 1 point |

The ICH score also is used in conjugate to the Functional Outcome in Patients with Primary Intracerebral Hemorrhage Score to predict a patient's functional independence at 90 days after ICH. The higher the score, the higher chance of functional independence.[48]

| | |
|---|---|
| ICH volume | < 30 mL (4 points), 30-60 mL (2 points), and > 60 mL (0 points) |
| Age | < 70 years (2 points), 70-79 years (1 point), and ≥ 80 years (zero points) |
| ICH location | Lobar (2 points), deep (1 point), infratentorial (0 points) |
| GCS | ≥ 9 (2 points), < 9 (0 points) |
| Pre-ICH cognitive impairment | No (1 point), yes (0 points) |

A systematic review including studies of patients after ICH estimated that between 12% and 39% of patients will achieve independent function.[49]

 What is the most important thing Susan can do to prevent her from having another ICH?

Uncontrolled hypertension is the most important risk factor for recurrent hemorrhage. Only about 5% of patients will have a recurrent ICH. The goal blood pressure is lower than 140/90. There appears to be a possible link between low low-density lipoprotein (LDL) cholesterol and risk of ICH. One study found that lower LDH cholesterol was predictive of early hematoma growth, neurological deteriorations, and 3-month mortality.[50] But there is no evidence that statins increase the risk of ICH.[51] Diet and exercise are important, but uncontrolled hypertension is the most important risk factor for recurrent ICH.

# Epidemiology

## *Stroke*

Stroke represents the most common life-threatening neurological condition and is the leading preventable cause of disability.[52] Every 40 seconds someone in the United Sates has a stroke.[52] It is the second-leading cause of death globally and fifth leading cause of death in the United States (after heart disease, cancer, chronic respiratory disease, and accidents), affecting approximately 6.3 million adults.[18-20] Cardiovascular diseases in general claim more lives than all forms of cancer combined.[52] The number of deaths from stroke per year in the United States is around 133,000, equating to nearly 42 deaths per 100,000 people.[18] Mortality varies and is based on race, age, and sex, with African American men having the highest risk.[52] Strokes are predicted to more than double in the next 20 years, with the highest increase, 5.1%, predicted for Americans between the ages of 45 and 64 years.[53] The cost of treatment for strokes is about $183 billion per year, with cost of loss of productivity at about $56 billion. It is predicted that Hispanic men will have the biggest increase in prevalence between now and 2030; the cost of treating strokes in Hispanic women is expected to triple during the same time period.[53]

There are multiple stroke risk scores that can help risk stratify patients presenting with strokes to provide insights into the likelihood of poor recovery.[12,54] Modifiable risk factors for stroke include hypertension, smoking, dyslipidemia, diabetes, atrial fibrillation, and physical inactivity.[55] Genetic factors also play an important role in stroke pathogenesis. Ischemic strokes either result from embolism, thrombosis, or systemic hypoperfusion, and there are multiple underlying causes of each. Hemorrhagic strokes normally result from a rupture of small vessel or aneurysm into the brain with etiologies ranging from hypertension, trauma, medications, vascular malformation, and amyloid angiopathy to bleeding diatheses.[55]

## *Movement Disorders (Parkinson's Disease)*

PD is the second most common neurodegenerative disease after AD.[25] It affects approximately 0.3% of the general population aged 40 years and older, with a steady rise in incidence between the ages of 70 and 79 years.[56,57] This equates to a prevalence of about 7.5 million people worldwide with increased prevalence with age. The mean age of onset is about 60 to 65 years. With the aging of the world's population, it is estimated that the prevalence will increase to 9 million people by 2030. The estimated incidence is about 10 per 100,000 per year.[58] The hallmark pathological features of PD are the depletion of dopamine caused by degeneration of neurons in the substantia nigra pars compacta, reduced striatal dopamine, and presence of Lewy bodies, which contain alpha synuclein. This leads to disruptions in connections between the thalamus and motor cortex causing parkinsonian symptoms.[25,57] Some studies suggest that the progression of Lewy bodies pathology is from the peripheral autonomic nervous system, to the olfactory system, to the dorsal motor nucleus of the vagus nerve of the lower brainstem, and then it spreads in a predictable manner to the upper brain stem and cerebral hemispheres (Braak Staging).[25,59] Epidemiologic studies on risk factors for PD have conclusively shown that age and family history are important risk factors, while smoking is associated with decreased risk.[60,61] Some studies suggest that men have a higher risk of developing PD than women.[56]

### Demyelinating Disorders (Multiple Sclerosis)

MS is a major cause of permanent disability among young adults, with onset typically in the 20s or 30s. The incidence and prevalence of MS varies dramatically based on geographic location and sex, with higher incidence in women and in locations such as northern Europe, northern United States, and Canada.[62-65] The cause of MS is unknown. Even though MS is thought to be autoimmune mediated, the specific antigen(s) hasn't been identified. However, there are numerous genetic and environmental factors thought to contribute to the risk, including family history, smoking, obesity, amount of sun exposure/vitamin D, and Epstein-Barr virus infection. The Multiple Sclerosis Foundation estimates that more than 400,000 people in the United States and about 2.5 million people around the world have MS. This equates to about 200 new cases each week in the United States.[66] The direct and indirect costs of MS in the United States range from $8,528 to $54,244 per patient per year.[67] There are four main types of MS: clinically isolated syndrome (CIS), relapsing-remitting (RRMS), secondary progressive (SPMS), and primary progressive (PPMS), with RRMS being the most common.[68]

### Neuromuscular Disorders (Amyotrophic Lateral Sclerosis)

ALS is a progressive motor neuron disorder with neural loss in the motor cortex, brain stem, and spinal cord. The estimated incidence is about two cases per 100,000, and prevalence ranges from 2.7 to 7.4 per 100,000.[69-71] This equates to about 7,000 new cases each year in the United States and about 500,000 who will develop this disease over their lifetime.[72] The incidence increases with each decade of age (especially after age 40 years), peaks around age 74 years, and then declines.[69] Most cases are sporadic or acquired with only about 10% of cases being inherited. Some familial cases have been linked to mutations in the superoxide dismutase-1 gene. There have been more than 40 ALS-associated genes identified.[72] There are occupational exposures and environmental toxins that appear to be risk factors for ALS.[73] There also appears to be a higher frequency in men younger than 70 years of age, but prevalence is similar in men and women after the age of 70.

Geographic clusters of ALS have occurred, with higher prevalence in the western Pacific, especially in Guam.[74] Also, military personnel appear to have an increased risk of ALS.[75] There have been multiple studies looking at additional risk factors, but thus far these have been inconclusive. The exact etiology of ALS is unknown, with multiple proposed mechanisms including abnormal ribonucleic acid (RNA) processing, mitochondrial dysfunction, viral infections, and others.[72] There also appears to be a link between ALS and frontotemporal dysfunction.[76]

### Jamel

Jamel is a 53-year-old man who is being evaluated in your clinic. He tells you that about 5 months ago he noticed he started having a tremor. The tremor is located in both of his hands and occurs at rest. He has past medical history of type 2 diabetes, hypertension, and chronic kidney disease. Medications include insulin glargine, insulin lispro, lisinopril, hydrochlorothiazide, and prochlorperazine. On exam he has decreased pedal pulses. He appears to have some speech difficulties. Mental status is normal. Cranial nerve function is normal, although a paucity of facial expression is noted. Movements are slow, and there is bilateral upper and lower extremity rigidity. Sensory exam reveals distal sensory loss. He has 4-Hz resting tremor in both upper extremities, along with a postural tremor and stooped posture.

 Which diagnoses should be considered at this time?

Drug-induced parkinsonism is the most likely diagnosis. This disorder is often secondary to neuroleptic medications but also can occur with any dopamine-blocking medication, including prochlorperazine and metoclopramide. Establishing the diagnosis of drug-induced parkinsonism is essential because stopping the medication can reverse or improve parkinsonian features. Sixty percent will recover within 2 months after discontinuation of the offending drug (although it may take as long as 2 years). Drug-induced parkinsonism is more prevalent in older adults and twice as common in women. It also is important to monitor this patient closely because sometimes drug-induced parkinsonism unmasks underlying early stages of PD.[77]

PD should be considered but is unlikely in this patient given the presence of bilateral tremor, rigidity, and postural tremor. Moreover, Jamel is taking a medication known to cause parkinsonism.

The patient does not have any cognitive problems, thus dementia of Lewy body is unlikely. Multiple-system atrophy should be considered, but even in an early stage, patients typically lack a tremor and normally present with cerebellar and autonomic signs and symptoms.

 What signs and symptoms are consistent with PD in this scenario?

The hallmark PD features are unilateral resting tremor, rigidity, bradykinesia, and postural instability. In more advance stages of the disease, patients will have cogwheel rigidity, akinesia, masked face, drooling, and inarticulate speech. Patients also may have autonomic dysfunctions. If you are seeing early falls and limited eye movements, you should consider progressive supranuclear palsy. If you are seeing ataxia and urinary incontinence, you should consider multiple-system atrophy. If you are seeing leg weakness and spasticity, ALS should be considered. If you are seeing cognitive impairment and irregular dance-like movements, consider HD.

## Disease Trajectory and Prognosis

### Stroke

The onset of a stroke is sudden and abrupt and typically follows a disease trajectory of rapid decline from normal baseline. Stroke evolution can lead to death, coma, or persistent vegetative state, or it can improve with or without disabilities.[12] Stroke continues to remain a major cause of death and disability despite advances in diagnosis and treatments. It is estimated that about one-fourth of stroke patients will die within the first 12 months, another third will have permanent disabilities, and the remaining generally become functionally independent after a couple of months with or without mild disabilities.[78,79] Age can have a significant impact on these rates.[80] Studies also have shown evidence of long-term and linear decline in functional status after a stroke for patients on Medicaid or who lack medical insurance, possibly secondary to poor healthcare access.[81] Decline can be three times greater for these patients.

Geographic location also appears to play a role. Higher stroke rates exist in the southeastern United States (the so-called stroke belt),[82] especially along the coasts of Georgia and the Carolinas (the so-called stroke buckle). Strokes are the second-leading global cause of death and fifth leading cause of death in the United States. It is estimated that worldwide 30-day mortality after ischemic stroke is between 16% and 23%.[19,83] Hemorrhagic strokes are associated with higher morbidity and mortality rates, with a 1-month mortality rate of 30% to 52%. Higher percentages are seen in patients with aneurysmal subarachnoid hemorrhages.[84,85] Because of the high rates of disability after a stroke, early stroke rehabilitation is paramount.

Decision-making capacity may also become impaired after a stroke, emphasizing the importance of early goals-of-care discussions and advance care planning with patients. At the onset, it is important for providers to support patients and family members given the unexpected and sometimes unpredictable nature that follows a stroke. It is also important to address this uncertainty when communicating to be able to establish realistic goals of care.

There are multiple prognostic tools available to help providers predict who will likely have poor neurological outcomes after a stroke. The National Institutes of Health Stroke Scale (NIHSS) is one of the most reliable prognostic tools to use after an ischemic stroke.[86] Additional prognostic tools include the ASTRAL score,[87] DRAGON score,[88] ISCORE,[89] and Plan score.[90] For hemorrhage strokes, there is the Glasgow Coma Scale (GCS), Hunt-Hess Grade

Scale, and World Federation of Neurologic Surgeons Scale, which is specifically used for sub-arachnoid hemorrhage. The intracerebral hemorrhage (ICH) score and Functional Outcome in Patients With Primary Intracerebral Hemorrhage (FUNC) score assess in cases of intracere-bral hemorrhage.[47,48] Poor prognostic factors include

- coma
- loss of brain-stem reflexes
- midline shift or herniation
- high NIHSS score (stroke severity)
- advanced age
- greater number of comorbidities (especially hypertension, diabetes, coronary artery disease, peripheral artery disease/peripheral vascular disease, and cognitive impairment)
- high prestroke disability scores
- stroke-related complications (eg, hemiplegia, urinary incontinence, gaze paresis, dysphagia)
- type of stroke (hemorrhagic worse than ischemic)
- presence of prestroke cognitive impairment
- low GCS score
- need for mechanical ventilation
- basilar artery occlusion with coma
- size, volume, and location of the infarction.[54,91-97]

The stroke severity can be judged clinically based on neurological exam and by the size and location of the infarction on MRI or computed tomography (CT). One study showed that 72 hours after an ischemic stroke, the infarct volume was an independent predictor of 90-day disability rates along with age and NIHSS.[96] Body mass index (BMI) is inversely related to stroke prognosis. The American Academy of Neurology issued guidelines in 2010 on the determination of brain death, which included the presence of irreversible coma, lack of brain-stem reflexes, no brain-generated response to external stimuli, and positive apnea test, although there are large variations among hospital policies.[98] The most common serious complications after a stroke include infection (especially pneumonia and urinary tract), respiratory failure necessitating mechanical ventilation, falls, pressure sores, pain, depression, heart failure, cardiac arrest, deep vein thrombosis/pulmonary embolism, and gastrointestinal bleed.[99,100] The rates of recurrent strokes, myocardial infarction, and death increase during the first 4 years after hospitalization for an acute stroke.[101] It is estimated that about 25% of patients will have an additional stroke within the first 5 years.

The greatest proportion of a patient's recovery time is in the first 3 to 6 months. Return of hand and arm function is a particularly positive prognostic marker. It is estimated that about 25% of patients will have minor disabilities, and about 40% will have moderate to severe disabilities after a stroke. Those patients with persistent neurological deficits at 6 months after a stroke can experience hemiparesis and cognitive deficits (about 40%); hemianopia, aphasia, dysphagia, or sensory deficits (about 20%); depression, gait abnormalities, bladder incontinence, and social disability (about 30%); and institutionalization (about 25%).[80] There are multiple disability scales that can be used, including Barthel Index, modified Rankin Scale, the Functional Independence Measure, and instrumental activities of daily living (IADLs).[84,102] Thus, given the high morbidity and mortality associated with acute strokes, many of these patients and family members will have specialized palliative care needs.

## Parkinson's Disease

PD is a chronic progressive disease with a course that spans years to decades. Patients develop motor and nonmotor symptoms as the disease progresses due to neurodegeneration in dopaminergic and nondopaminergic structures.[103] In recent decades there have been many advances in symptomatic treatment of PD, but there is no established therapy that will halt or slow the progression of this disease in a meaningful way.

Life expectancy is varied and often depends on age of onset and presence of dementia and other comorbidities. The average age of onset is 60 years. Median survival ranges from 6 to 22 years.[104,105] Increasing age and presence of dementia or cognitive decline are associated with increased risk of mortality. Severity of axial symptoms (balance, gait, postural dysfunction) also is an important prognostic indicator. In 2016 Velseboer and colleagues developed a prognostic model—patients with greater age, higher Unified Parkinson's Disease Rating Scale (UPDRS) motor examination axial score, and a lower animal fluency score were all associated with a higher probability of an unfavorable outcome (such as disability, dementia, and death).[106] **Table 20** lists average life expectancies based on age of disease onset.[107] The natural progression of PD following Hoehn and Yahr's five major stages is described in **Table 21**; some patients will die before progressing through all stages. A modified scale also exists.[108] The UPDRS scale is more comprehensive than the Hoehn and Yahr scale. It takes into account cognitive difficulties, ability to carry out daily activities, behavior, mood, and treatment complications along with movement symptoms. During the early stages of disease, the focus is shifted to minimize dyskinesia, decrease occurrences of motor and nonmotor on-off symptoms, and maximize independence.[109] In the later stages of PD, the role of palliative care expands as patients and family members are greatly impacted by the high symptom burden, especially of nonmotor symptoms during later stages. The National Parkinson's Foundation recommends palliative care involvement if patients have the following: stage 3 or higher, dementia, psychosis, or significant caregiver strain.[110] There is also the MacMahon and Thomas 4-stage model of PD:

- stage 1: diagnosis (last about 2 years)
- stage 2: maintenance (last about 6 years)
- stage 3: complex (last about 5 years)
- stage 4: palliative (last about 2.2 years).[111]

## Table 20. Life Expectancy in Parkinson's Disease

| Age of Onset (Years) | Average Life Expectancy (Years) |
|---|---|
| 25-39 | 38-49 |
| 40-59 | 30 |
| 50-59 | 20 |
| 60-64 | 15 |
| ≥ 65 | 5-10 |

## Table 21. Stages of Parkinson's Disease

| | |
|---|---|
| Stage 1 | Typically the first 3 years of the disease, when patients demonstrate unilateral disease with minimal functional impairment. Because the symptoms are not very pronounced, this stage often goes underdiagnosed. Patients will start having slowing of movements, unilateral resting tremor, impaired coordination, and some rigidity. |
| Stage 2 | Bilateral involvement develops years after onset. Signs and symptoms consist of bilateral loss of facial expression, decreased blinking, speech abnormalities, worsening rigidity, gait abnormalities, and postural abnormalities without impairments in balance. Most patients during this stage are still independent in activities of daily living (ADLs). |
| Stage 3 | Patients develop impairments in balance and postural reflexes and increased falls, along with significant slowing of body movements. |
| Stage 4 | Patients develop severe impairments and are no longer able to function independently in all ADLs, requiring the use of a walker and an inability to live alone. Significant rigidity and bradykinesia exist. |
| Stage 5 | Patients generally require the use of a wheelchair because their ability to transfer from a chair becomes remarkably impaired. Patients will have problems falling when standing or turning, increased freezing episodes, dysphagia, dysarthria, and impaired coordination. This often is considered the cachectic stage. At this stage, hospice should be considered and discussed. |

The "palliative phase" has been defined by waning response to dopaminergic agents and presence of cognitive decline.[112,113] This phase typically last about 2.2 years.[111]

Nonmotor complications in late stages of PD consist of dementia, hallucinations/psychosis, depression, anxiety, apathy, fatigue, olfactory dysfunction, dysregulation of blood pressure, autonomic dysfunction, bowel and bladder problems, constipation, and sleep disturbances.[114-116] It is estimated that about 40% of patients with PD will develop dementia.[117] Most patients with

PD typically will die from aspiration pneumonia. The prolonged course of PD, in conjunction with increasing functional impairment and symptom burden, necessitates a careful assessment of care goals along with early advance care planning.

## Multiple Sclerosis

MS is a chronic condition characterized by recurrent episodes of demyelination in the CNS. The clinical course is highly variable, and QOL often is greatly impacted. There are several clinical subtypes, which include CIS, RRMS, SPMS, and PPMS.[68] The phenotypes are modified based on disease progression and disease activity. MS typically starts with a clinical attack in about 85% of patients.[20,118] **Table 22** describes the main clinical subtypes and their disease courses, and **Figure 3** illustrates the disease trajectories of RRMS, SPMS, and PPMS, respectively.[68,119]

The course of MS often is described in two phases: the early phase, which is often modifiable with treatment (immunomodulation) and during which disability is often minor,[122] and the late phase, in which there is irreversible neurodegeneration, causing multiple complications and a variety of symptoms (eg, fatigue, spasticity, palsies, dysphagia, dysarthria, pain, psychosocial distress). Thus, in the later stage, treatment becomes challenging, and in severe MS, a wide range of healthcare specialists often are needed.[122]

The most common symptoms include weakness or numbness, optic neuritis, tremor or ataxic gait, double vision, dysarthria, dizziness, and fatigue. Poor prognosis factors include involvement in more than one neurological system at onset, diagnosis of PPMS, high number of attacks within the first few years after onset, high disability rating (eg, Kurtzke disability scale) at 5 years after onset, African American race, and older age at onset.[118] Permanent disability can take many forms and is highly variable and includes ataxia, vision loss, and dementia, but it most commonly involves gait abnormalities.

Fifteen to 25 years after diagnosis, many patients will require an assistive device to ambulate (eg, cane); about 20% will be bed bound or institutionalized.[118] It is estimated that as many as one-third of patients will never develop any permanent disabilities. Mortality in patients with MS is variable, but it appears that life expectancy is reduced by about 7 to 14 years. For about 50% of patients, MS is the main cause of death.[123] Most patients with MS will die from the same conditions as the general population, but they do have higher rates of cardiovascular disease, suicide, and infections.[124,125] The risk of suicide is about two times higher in those with MS than the general population (one study showed seven times higher than the general population[126]).[125,127] Thus, given the unpredictability of MS, it can be a very devastating disease, and it is very important to have early goals of care discussions along with assessment and management of psychological symptoms in addition to typical treatment modalities.

## Amyotrophic Lateral Sclerosis

ALS is a progressive neurodegenerative disease with loss of bulbar and limb function. The median survival of patients with ALS from time of onset ranges from 20 to 48 months. Most

## Table 22. Clinical Subtypes and Disease Courses of Multiple Sclerosis

| Clinical Subtype | Disease Course |
|---|---|
| Clinically isolated syndrome (CIS) | CIS is the first attack (eg, optic neuritis, transverse myelitis) that is consistent with inflammatory demyelination but doesn't meet the criteria yet for the diagnosis of MS because there needs to be dissemination that occurs at different times and in different locations.[118] This episode must last for at least 24 hours. The 2010 revisions to the McDonald MS diagnostic criteria allow some patients with a single clinical episode to be diagnosed with MS based on the specific findings in the MRI that show episodes of damage in different locations along with indications of active inflammation.[43] Most patients are diagnosed between the ages of 20 and 40 years, with median age of 30 years.[119] |
| | For patients with CIS who have an abnormal MRI, about 60% will progress to MS; for those with normal MRI, only about 20% will progress to MS.[118] After there is evidence of "dissemination in time" either by second attack or lesions seen on MRI, the diagnosis of relapsing-remitting MS is confirmed. |
| Relapsing-remitting MS (RRMS) | RRMS is characterized by a clearly defined new attack after the initial attack of CIS as discussed above, followed by periods of partial or complete recovery (remissions). During remissions, all symptoms may disappear, although some may become permanent. However, there is no apparent progression of disease during remissions. This type of MS accounts for approximately 85%-90% of cases.[68,119,120] |
| | Over time, the frequency of the attacks increases and degree of recovery from an individual relapse declines.[20] Thus, the risk of residual neurological impairment increases after each attack as the disease progresses. The course is very heterogeneous; early in the disease course, the attack can occur every 12-14 months, or patients can have several attacks during the first year or maintain remission for years.[118] |
| | About two-thirds of patients with RRMS will convert to secondary progressive MS after about 10-20 years.[118] Typically this is seen as gradual worsening gait disorder. |
| Secondary progressive MS (SPMS) | SPMS typically is diagnosed retrospectively after a history of gradual worsening in patients with RRMS with or without occasional relapses, minor remissions, and plateaus.[68,119] Over time, patients stop having remissions and begin to steadily worsen. The transition from RRMS to SPMS as stated above often occurs after about 10-20 years.[119,121] |

*Continued on page 124*

**Table 22. Clinical Subtypes and Disease Courses of Multiple Sclerosis** *(continued)*

| Clinical Subtype | Disease Course |
|---|---|
| Primary progressive MS (PPMS) | PPMS is characterized more as a gradual worsening of disease than distinct attacks (no relapses or remissions). This occurs in about 10%-15% of patients with MS. This can be challenging to diagnose. It is diagnosed primarily clinically, but serial MRIs and laboratory studies, including cerebrospinal fluid and evoked potentials, can help support the diagnosis.[68,119] This subtype of MS is extremely difficult for patients because there are no signs of remission, and their condition continues to worsen despite treatment. Symptoms become more grueling to manage, greatly impacting their QOL and functional ability. PPMS typically develops later in life (fifth or sixth decade) and is the most severe subtype of MS because it will follow a course similar to secondary progressive at the time of diagnosis.[118] |

**Figure 3. Disease and Disability Trajectories for Subtypes of Multiple Sclerosis[119]**

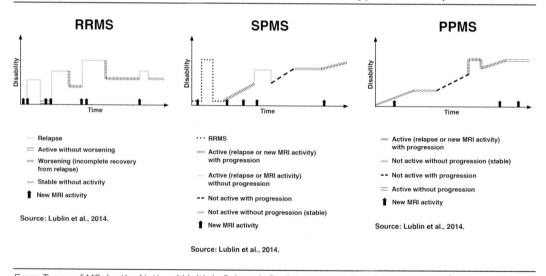

*From Types of MS, by the National Multiple Sclerosis Society, www.nationalmssociety.org/What-is-MS/Types-of-MS, Accessed June 29, 2017. © National Multiple Sclerosis Society. Reproduced with permission.*

patients will die from respiratory failure within 3 to 5 years of symptom onset; of the remaining patients, about 10% will survive as long as 8 to 10 years after onset.[128] The initial symptoms typically are painless, such as weakness, atrophy, and fasciculation beginning in either an arm or leg.[20,128] Patients will not have pain, sensory loss, or impairments in bowel or bladder function as their chief complaint; these symptoms may develop later in the disease course, but it is unclear if they are related to ALS. Also typically seen are upper motor neuron signs of hyperflexia and extensor plantar responses. It is estimated that about 20% to 30% will have bulbar onset ALS, marked by slurred speech, emotional lability, and difficulty swallowing. About 5% of patients will have respiratory onset disease. As the disease progresses, patients will develop weight loss, malnutrition, and respiratory insufficiency eventually requiring ventilator support. About 15% of patients will develop frontotemporal dementia and 20% executive impairment. Executive dysfunction is often seen as impaired judgment and impulsivity and is a strong negative prognostic factor. The site of onset has prognostic importance; onset in limbs carries a better prognosis than in the bulbar region, and lower-limb onset has a better prognosis than upper-limb onset. The worse prognosis appears in respiratory onset. **Table 23** lists factors thought to be associated with a poorer prognosis in ALS.[128-131] Given the poor prognosis and impact on QOL, a multidisciplinary management approach is needed for patients with ALS with a strong focus on symptom management and goals of care. Palliative care can play an integral role in the management of ALS at diagnosis, and hospice services are beneficial near the end of life.

## Table 23. Poor Prognostic Indicators in Amyotrophic Lateral Sclerosis

| | |
|---|---|
| Age > 65 years | Bulbar or respiratory onset disease |
| Malnutrition (BMI < 25) | High levels of psychological distress |
| Frontal temporal dementia | Forced vital capacity < 50% |
| Sniff nasal inspiratory pressure < 40 cm $H_2O$ | Short interval from first symptom to diagnosis |

## Clinical Situation

### Mikaya

Mikaya is a 26-year-old woman who presents to your office after a 1-week history of numbness in her left leg. She has no significant past medical history and takes no medications. On further questioning, she does tell you that about 1 year ago she had a 2-week episode of diplopia and vertigo (which completely resolved). On physical exam, vitals are normal. She has extensor plantar response on the left. When testing for vibration, sensation is mildly impaired in both feet, and she has decreased pain sensation on her left leg. Laboratory test results are all normal. MRI of her brain shows a small periventricular white matter lesion.

 What is the appropriate next step in the management of Mikaya's symptoms?

This patient should undergo a lumbar puncture. There is a high suspicion that this patient has MS given her age, prior neurological event, abnormal neurological findings on exam, and abnormal MRI. However, these are insufficient to confirm that multiple regions of the CNS are affected at different times (dissemination in time and space). Thus, doing a lumbar puncture and showing oligoclonal bands or elevated IgG index will help confirm the diagnosis. An electroencephalogram (EEG) and MRA would not help confirm that different parts of the CNS are affected. Antibody testing (eg, myelin basic protein) may reveal that antibodies are present, but testing is not used to diagnosis MS.

 You follow up with Mikaya 3 months later. She currently is asymptomatic. She has completely recovered from her neurological attack 3 months ago. What type of MS does this patient most likely have?

She most likely has RRMS. She had two attacks at different times and has recovered from those events. Eighty-five percent of patients will have this type of MS. PPMS, which occurs in about 15% of patients, is defined as gradual worsening of neurological function over more than 1 year without recovery. SPMS occurs years after a patient has RRMS. Median time to conversion is about 10 to 15 years. The conversion to SPMS will occur in about 60% of patients with RRMS.

 What factor (or factors) are associated with a better prognosis for a patient with MS?

The prognosis for men with MS appears to be worse than for women. Onset of disease after the age of 40 years, cerebellar symptoms, more than two attacks in 2 years, poor recovery after an exacerbation, disability within 5 years, and impaired motor symptoms at onset are all associated with a poorer prognosis. Prognosticating is very difficult in MS, but identifying factors associated with a worse prognosis may help.[132,133]

 How might we measure disability in patients with MS?

Utilizing the Expanded Disability Status Scale (EDSS), a higher score is associated with poorer prognosis. Studies have shown a correlation between the number of risk factors and EDSS score. However, the EDSS captures cognitive impairment poorly. It also is a nonlinear ordinal scale and heavily dependent on mobility. It is insensitive to small changes within a patient. Scores of 0.0 to 4.5 refer to patients fully ambulatory, and scores of 5.0 to 9.5 are defined by the impairment in ambulation. A score of 10 is associated with death from MS.

 **What other comorbidities should we be concerned with for this patient?**

It is very important to screen Mikaya for depression because up to two-thirds of patients with MS have it. They also have a higher rate of suicide than the general population. It also is important to screen for fatigue because up to 78% of patients will report this symptom. It is recommended to first screen for depression because depression can cause fatigue. Cognitive impairment can occur in patients with MS, but only about 5% of patients will have dementia. Mild cognitive impairment occurs in up to 70% of patients, but, for most, cognitive dysfunction does not impact daily function.[134] Dysphagia can also occur in MS, but it is more frequently found in advanced disease.

## Management, Symptom Assessment, and Control

### Stroke

The management of acute stroke will depend on the etiology and the timing from the onset of symptoms to the patient's presentation at the hospital. In acute ischemic strokes, patients who present to the hospital less than 4.5 hours from the onset of symptoms and who do not have any exclusionary criteria can be candidates for intravenous thrombolytic therapy (eg, alteplase, tenecteplase).[135] Strict blood pressure control is important before and 24 hours after thrombolytic therapy. The most feared complication after thrombolytic therapy is intracerebral hemorrhage, which occurs in about 5% to 7% of patients.[136,137] Endovascular therapy approaches include endovascular pharmacological thrombolysis, mechanical and aspiration thrombectomy, the use of a guidewire or microcatheter to manipulate the clot, and stent retriever technology. Patients who are not candidates for intravenous thrombolysis or mechanical thrombectomy are treated with antiplatelet agents, typically aspirin. In addition, good glucose control, management of dehydration, and statin therapy are important. Options for secondary stroke prevention include aspirin, clopidogrel, or aspirin/extended-release dipyridamole. In patients with underlying atrial fibrillations, long-term therapy consists of warfarin, direct thrombin inhibitor (dabigatran), or direct factor Xa inhibitors (rivaroxaban, apixaban).[138]

For patients with ICH, treatment will depend on etiology. The most common primary causes of ICH are hypertension, medications (especially antiplatelet, anticoagulant, and thrombolytic drugs), and cerebral amyloid angiopathy. If the ICH is secondarily to heparin, protamine sulfate is used. If secondary to warfarin, vitamin K and fresh frozen plasma (FFP) are used. If secondary to thrombolytic therapy, cryoprecipitate is used. If secondary to dabigatran, idarucizumab (praxbind) can be used as a reversal agent.[139] There is no reversal agent for direct factor Xa inhibitors, but typically unactivated 4-factor-prothrombin complex concentrate is used.[140] For patients with cerebellar hemorrhage greater than 3 cm with deteriorating neurological symptoms or brain-stem compression or hydrocephalus, emergent surgical evacuation is indicated.[141] Patients with aneurysmal subarachnoid hemorrhage have very high mortality rates—45% in 1 month. About 10% will die prior to reaching the hospital.[142] Treatment consists of aneurysm repair (surgical clipping or endovascular coiling), discontinuation of any antithrombotic medication, close monitoring of intracranial pressure, good blood pressure control, and management of any complications (vasospasm, hydrocephalus, hyponatremia, seizures, or rebleeding).

Poststroke management includes rehabilitation, control of risk factors, and symptom and psychological management. A focus on trying to improve QOL for patients after a stroke is essential. About one-third of patients will have communication difficulties after a stroke, which can make assessment challenging. See **Table 24** for common symptoms and management after stroke.

### Parkinson's Disease

Management of PD can be categorized by motor versus nonmotor symptoms. The main motor symptoms are tremor, rigidity, bradykinesia, and postural instability. **Table 25** describes treatment approaches for the management of common motor symptoms. Deep brain stimulators also are used to help with tremor, the on/off fluctuations, and dyskinesia in patients with intractable symptoms. Deep brain stimulators typically are placed in either the subthalamic nucleus or internal globus pallidus.[154] Hardware complications can occur (about 1%-4%), the most common being electrode/wire replacement, device dysfunction, infection, or migrations.[155] In addition, surgical and stimulation-related complications (eg, dysarthria, weight gain, depression/psychosis, eyelid apraxia) can occur, as well as cognitive and behavioral complications, particularly an increased risk of suicide.[156]

The main nonmotor symptoms consist of dementia, hallucinations/psychosis, depression, anxiety, apathy, fatigue, olfactory dysfunction, gastrointestinal problems (particularly constipation), dysregulation of blood pressure/autonomic dysfunction, bowel and bladder problems, early satiety, hyperhidrosis, seborrhea, sexual dysfunction, sensory problems (pain, tingling, burning), and sleep disturbances. Mixed motor and nonmotor symptoms include drooling (sialorrhea) and speech and swallowing problems. The Edmonton Symptom Assessment System–PD assesses symptom burden.[110] Typically anosmia, sleep disorders, and autonomic dysfunction occur early in the disease course, then motor symptoms. Later in the disease course, emotional and cognitive problems may develop. The nonmotor symptoms can cause more disability in patients with PD than the classic motor features. Up to 90% of patients with PD will experience at least one nonmotor symptom, with up to 50% of patients having depression.[157] The Beck Depression Inventory-I, Hamilton Depression Rating Scale, or Montgomery

## Table 24. Common Symptoms After Stroke

| Symptom | Incidence | Assessment Tools | Management |
|---|---|---|---|
| Poststroke depression (PSD) and emotional lability | About 30% of patients will have PSD. About 2% will have pseudobulbar affect. | PHQ-2 or PHQ-9, BDI, HAM-D, HADS, clinical global impression tool[143] | PSD: mainstay treatment is SSRIs[144] Emotional lability: dextromethorphan/quinidine[144] |
| Anxiety | About 20% | HAM-A, GAI, HADS | SSRIs or SNRIs. Benzodiazepines should be used only in severe cases or for those with limited life span. |
| Delirium | 10%-48% | CAM-ICU, DRS, 3D-CAM, 4AT | Behavioral modifications, management of any identifiable causes, antipsychotics (only in those with hyperactive delirium who are risk to self or others) |
| Dysphagia | 20%-50% | Swallowing evaluation bedside or VFS, FEES | Rehab, chin tuck maneuver, specialized diet. NG tube and PEG tube have not been shown to decrease aspiration/dysphagia but can help improve nutritional status. |
| Pain | Central poststroke pain (CPSP): about 12% of patients[144] Hemiplegic shoulder pain (HSP): ranges from 48% to 84%[144] | Abbey Pain Scale,[145] Vertical VAS, FPS, NRS, DOLOPLUS-2, nociception coma scale[146] | CPSP: amitriptyline, lamotrigine[147] HSP: electrical stimulation, physical therapy, NSAIDS, massage, ice/heat, strapping/sling, botulinum toxin, denervation procedure, or acupuncture[148] |
| Poststroke spasticity (PSS) | About 30%[144] | Modified Ashworth Scale, Tardieu Scale, Carer Burden Scale, Disability Assessment Scale[149] | Botulinum injection, physical therapy, splints/orthoses, electrical stimulation, and antispastic agents[149] |
| Fatigue | About 50%[144] | FSMC, Fatigue Severity Scale, Modified Fatigue Impact Scale,[150] the Brief Fatigue Inventory,[151] and others | Modafinil,[152] amantadine, methylphenidate |

Continued on page 130

**Table 24. Common Symptoms After Stroke** *(continued)*

| Symptom | Incidence | Assessment Tools | Management |
|---|---|---|---|
| Urinary incontinence: incomplete emptying (overflow), urge or stress incontinence | 50% during initial hospitalization; 20% urinary incontinence at 6 months[144] | History, physical exam, urodynamic testing, postvoid residual, bladder stress test | Nonpharmacological: weight loss, dietary changes, bladder training, biofeedback, pelvic floor exercises, incontinence pads, indwelling catheters, external urinary catheters<br><br>Pharmacological: alpha blockers, antimuscarinic drugs, SNRIs<br><br>Surgical treatment is considered when symptom is unresponsive to medical management. |
| Fecal incontinence | 10% fecal incontinence at 6 months[144] | History, physical exam, anorectal manometry, endorectal ultrasound/MRI, defecography | Supportive care, medical therapy aimed at reducing stool frequency (bulking agents, antidiarrheal agents), biofeedback, injectable anal bulking agent, sacral nerve stimulation, and anal sphincteroplasty |
| Seizures/epilepsy | 5%-12%[153] | EEG, physical exam, MRI | Antiepileptic drugs are controversial.[153] |
| Sexual dysfunction | As high as 50% | History, hormonal lab tests | Counseling, medication review, depression screening<br><br>Safety and efficacy of medications for erectile dysfunction such as phosphodiesterase inhibitors (eg, sildenafil) after recent stroke is controversial. |
| Sleep disordered breathing | As high as 50% | Sleep study | Weight loss, CPAP/BiPAP |

*4AT, the 4 "As" Test; BDI, Beck Depression Inventory; BiPAP, bilevel positive airway pressure; CAM, Confusion Assessment Method; CPAP, continuous positive airway pressure; CT, computed tomography; DRS, Delirium Rating Scale; EEG, electroencephalogram; FEES, fiberoptic endoscopic evaluation of swallowing; FPS, faces pain scale; FSMC, Fatigue Scale for Motor and Cognitive Functions; GAI, Geriatric Anxiety Inventory scale; HAM-A, Hamilton Anxiety Rating Scale; HAM-D, Hamilton Depression Rating Scale; HADS, Hospital Anxiety and Depression Scale; NG, nasogastric; NRS, numeric rating scale; NSAIDS, nonsteroidal anti-inflammatory drugs; PEG, percutaneous endoscopic gastrostomy; PHQ, Patient Health Questionnaire; SNRI, serotonin-norepinephrine reuptake inhibitor; SSRI, selective serotonin reuptake inhibitor; VAS, visual analog scale; VFS, video fluoroscopic exam*

# Table 25. Symptomatic Therapy for Parkinson's Disease

| Drug | Dosing | Benefit | Common Side Effects |
|------|--------|---------|---------------------|
| **Levodopa:** *Abruptly stopping these drugs can cause neuroleptic malignant syndrome or akinetic crisis.* | | | |
| Carbidopa/levodopa (comes in many formularies and in combination with entacapone [Stavelo]) | Available tablets: 10/100 mg, 25/100 mg, 25/250 mg<br><br>Starting dose, 25/100 mg, one-half tablet two or three times daily with meals | Effective management of bradykinetic symptoms | Nausea, somnolence, dizziness, headaches, motor fluctuations (the wearing-off phenomenon), dyskinesia, dystonia, cramps, constipation, orthostatic hypotension |
| Duopa (enteral suspension of carbidopa/levodopa) | Infusion system into jejunal tube for 16 hours<br><br>Dosing will depend on patient's daily dose of levodopa. | Improves on/off fluctuations, decreases dyskinesia (does not improve tremor) | Complication of device<br><br>Same side effect profile as carbidopa/levodopa. Additional side effects are depression, edema, hypertension, infection. |
| Apomorphine | Starting dose 2 mg SC (max dose is 6 mg) | Improves "off" symptoms | Chest pain, drowsiness, dizziness, orthostatic hypotension, nausea, dyskinesia, falls, yawning |
| **Dopamine agents:** *Abruptly stopping these drugs can cause anxiety, panic attacks, depression, sweating, nausea, pain, fatigue, dizziness, and drug craving.* | | | |
| Pramipexole and ropinirole | Pramipexole starting dose 0.125 mg twice daily<br><br>Ropinirole starting dose 0.25 mg twice daily<br><br>Both also are available as sustained-released formations. | Effective management of bradykinetic symptoms and dyskinesia | Nausea, vomiting, sleepiness, orthostatic hypotension, confusion, hallucinations, peripheral edema, dopaminergic dysregulation syndrome (compulsive disorder), impulse control disorder |
| Rotigotine patch | Starting dose 2 mg every 24 hours | Same as pramipexole and ropinirole | Same as pramipexole and ropinirole |

*Continued on page 132*

## Table 25. Symptomatic Therapy for Parkinson's Disease *(continued)*

| Drug | Dosing | Benefit | Common Side Effects |
|------|--------|---------|---------------------|
| **Other** | | | |
| Amantadine | Starting dose 100 mg twice daily | Improves bradykinesia, rigidity, and tremor | Livedo reticularis, ankle edema, hallucinations, confusion, nightmares |
| **COMT Inhibitors** | | | |
| Entacapone | Starting dose 200 mg with each dose of levodopa | Decrease in motor fluctuations, decreases "off" symptoms | Diarrhea, discolored urine, dyskinesia, hallucinations, confusion, nausea, orthostatic hypotension |
| Tolcapone | Starting dose 100 mg twice daily | Same as entacapone | Same as entacapone, plus hepatotoxicity |
| **MAO-B Inhibitors** | | | |
| Rasagiline (Azilect) | Starting dose 0.5 mg daily | Decreased motor fluctuations ("off time"), better UPDRS scores | Nausea, headache, confusion, dyskinesia, psychiatric toxicities, orthostatic hypotension |
| Selegiline (eldepryl, zelapar) | 5 mg twice daily | Same as rasagiline | Same as rasagiline |
| **Anticholinergics** | | | |
| Trihexyphenidyl (Artane) | Starting dose 0.5 mg twice daily | Useful in young patients with tremor-predominant PD | Confusion, hallucinations, urinary retention, tachycardia, dizziness, constipation, nausea, blurry vision |

*COMT, catechol-O-methyl transferase; SC, subcutaneous; UPDRS, Unified Parkinson's Disease Rating Scale*

Asberg Depression Rating Scale should be used to screen for depression in PD.[157] No clear consensus exists on which antidepressant to use for patients with PD, but selective serotonin reuptake inhibitors (SSRIs) are commonly used to start, with close monitoring for worsening of motor symptoms and possible interactions with monoamine oxidase B (MAO-B) inhibitors (if used) causing serotonin syndrome.[158,159] Visual hallucinations and paranoid delusions are common—up to 40%.[160] Treatments can vary from dose adjustment of antiparkinsonian drugs to use of atypical neuroleptics (clozapine, quetiapine) or a selective serotonin 5-HT2A agonist (pimavanserin).[160] It is very important to limit the use of any antidopamine medications (eg, haldoperidol). Sadly there is no effective treatment available at this time to manage fatigue and daytime sleepiness, but trials of amantadine or methylphenidate are frequently considered.[160] Sialorrhea and drooling are common manifestations and can be treated with chewing gum or hard candy for mild symptoms or botulinum toxin injection, glycopyrrolate, or other anticholinergic medications (eg, hyoscyamine, atropine) for more severe symptoms. Rhinorrhea often is treated with ipratropium nasal spray, which seems to be effective. Pain is very common, even in early PD. Managing pain often requires a multidisciplinary approach and may include

- dopaminergic medications or botulinum injections (to help with levodopa-related dystonia)
- conservative or nonpharmacologic therapies
  - » physical and/or occupational therapies
  - » nonsteroidal anti-inflammatory drugs (NSAIDS)
  - » selective norepinephrine reuptake inhibitors (SNRI)
  - » electrotherapy stimulation
  - » muscle relaxants
- surgery (deep brain stimulation to help with dystonia)
- conventional therapies with opioids.[161]

Constipation also can be challenging, and small studies have shown benefits of lubiprostone and polyethylene glycol.[162] Management of cognitive impairment will depend on etiology as well as differentiating PD-related dementia from PD with Alzheimer's, PD with vascular dementia, and Lewy body dementia. PD-related dementia typically is treated with cholinesterase inhibitors, but close monitoring of side effects is needed, especially worsened tremor and nausea.[160] Because of the high percentage of nonmotor symptoms experienced by patients with PD, palliative care can play an integral role in improving QOL for this population.

## Multiple Sclerosis
### Disease-Modifying Therapies
The mainstay treatment for MS is disease-modifying therapy. Treatments depend on whether the patient has CIS, RRMS, SPMS, or PPMS. The main disease-modifying therapies can be found in **Table 26.** These treatments have been approved for RRMS but do not appear to be

## Table 26. Main Disease-Modifying Therapies for Multiple Sclerosis[163]

| Drug | Mechanism | Common Side Effects |
|---|---|---|
| Interferon beta preparations; beta-1a, beta-1b | Immunomodulatory | Flu-like symptoms, fatigue, depression, abnormal LFTs<br>Monitor CBCs and LFTs every 6 months |
| Glatiramer acetate | Immunomodulatory | Injection site reactions, dyspnea, panic attack–like syndrome |
| Natalizumab | Selective adhesion molecule inhibitor | Risk of progressive multifocal leukoencephalopathy, headaches, back pain, infusion reactions |
| Alemtuzumab | Monoclonal antibody to CD52 | ITP, infection, infusion reactions, autoimmune disorders |
| Mitoxantrone | Type II topoisomerase inhibitor | Cardiac toxicity, nausea and vomiting, heartburn, hair loss, immunosuppression |
| Dimethyl fumarate (oral) | Activate nuclear factor 2 (Nrf2) pathway | Flushing, GI symptoms |
| Teriflunomide (oral) | Immunomodulatory agent that inhibits pyrimidine synthesis | Headache, alopecia, GI symptoms, elevated ALT, infection |
| Fingolimod (oral) | Binds to sphingosine 1-phosphate receptors (blocks the lymphocytes' ability to emerge from lymph nodes) | Headache, infection, GI symptoms, elevated LFTs, cough, back pain, bradyarrhythmia |
| Corticosteroids | Immunomodulatory | Insomnia, flushing, metallic taste, fluid retention, electrolyte abnormalities, hyperglycemia |

*ALT, alanine aminotransferase; CBC, complete blood count; GI, gastrointestinal; ITP, idiopathic thrombocytopenic purpura; LFT, liver function test*

as effective in treating progressive forms of MS. The main treatments consist of fingolimod, azathioprine, cladribine, dalfampridine, glucocorticoids, cyclophosphamide, cyclosporine, interferons, methotrexate, mitoxantrone, natalizumab, rituximab, or simvastatin. Other, less commonly used immune-modulating treatments include stem-cell transplantation, intravenous immunoglobulin infusions, plasma exchange, and total lymphoid irradiation. The goals of all immunomodulatory or immunosuppressive therapies are to decrease relapse rates, reduce relapse severity, and decrease accumulation of lesions in the CNS. Most patients will continue preventive therapy their entire lives.[163] These therapies have shown to decrease risk of relapse by about one-third and to modestly slow the progression of the disease.[20] Most patients should be monitored for acute exacerbations and new CNS lesions by using the Expanded Disability Scale every 3 months and brain MRI every 12 months.[163] Patients with refractory disease often will be switched to a different agent to determine effectiveness.

### Treatment of Acute Exacerbation

Most acute flares of MS will have minimal impact on a patient's function; thus, treatment is not needed. If a patient does develop symptoms that impair function, such as loss of vision, motor symptoms, or balance/coordination problems, treatment with steroids is indicated. Methylprednisolone, 1 g per day for up to 5 days, or oral prednisone taper are the most common therapies used.[164] Small studies have looked at plasma exchange for patients who do not respond to glucocorticoid therapy, so this should be considered, especially in those with severe neurological deficits.[165] The most important thing to determine is whether the episode is a true MS relapse or an infection, which can be accomplished with a thorough history and physical exam along with a targeted workup.

### Symptomatic Treatment and General Health Care

Like many chronic diseases, patients with MS often have high symptom burden that should be assessed and managed to optimize QOL. Given the varied course of MS, there is a large variety of symptoms that range from fatigue and physical dysfunction (eg, spasticity, palsies, swallowing or speech problems) to pain, urinary symptoms, and spiritual and psychological distress (eg, depression).[122] Different scales are available to monitor symptoms, including the Palliative care Outcome Scale, expanded disability status scale, different QOL scales (eg, CAREQOL-MS), and caregiver burden scales (eg, Zarit Caregiver Burden Interview).

Fatigue is a very common symptom for people with MS, with rates up to 78%, and is exacerbated by heat and humidity.[166] Treatment options include amantadine, methylphenidate, 4-aminopyridine (fampridine), L-carnitine, selective serotonin reuptake inhibitors (SSRIs), aspirin, and modafinil.[167] Nonpharmacological treatments for fatigue for these patients include massage, exercise, cognitive-behavioral therapy, and nutritional consult.[168] It also is important to rule out possible causes or triggers of fatigue, such as hypothyroidism, anemia, sleep disorders, depression, pain, medications, and other medical conditions. Amantadine, 100 mg twice a day, has been studied in the treatment of fatigue, but there is insufficient evidence to make recommendations for its use at this time.[169] Some patients may respond to methylphenidate and modafinil; current studies are determining their efficacy.[170] Given the high rate of depression, SSRIs have also been used to treat underlying fatigue. A small randomized study has shown that the use of aspirin, 1,300 mg daily, appears to be modestly effective in treating fatigue, but larger trials are needed.[171] Rehabilitation interventions appear to have stronger and more significant effects on reducing the impact or severity of fatigue and should be considered.[170]

Almost two-thirds of patients with MS experience depression, and the risk of suicide is two times higher than in the general population.[125,127,172] Treatment should involve psychotherapy and pharmacotherapy. Data are limited on the pharmacological treatment of depression for patients with MS. A *Cochrane* review reported desipramine and paroxetine to have modest efficacy but with a high side-effect profile; further research is needed.[173]

Up to 40% of patients with MS will complain of pain, which typically is neuropathic in nature.[174] Treatment options include tricyclic antidepressants, anticonvulsants (gabapentin, pregabalin, carbamazeprine), SNRIs, physiotherapy, NSAIDs, acetaminophen, cannabinoids, and other agents.[174] For refractory symptoms, therapies such as radiofrequency rhizotomy can be considered. Spasticity is common and often can be painful. Treatment often consist of physical therapy (stretching) and oral antispasticity drugs (baclofen, tizanidine, dantrolene).[174,175] If symptoms are severe or refractory, a trial with botulinum toxin injection or intrathecal baclofen pump may be considered.

Urinary incontinence also is a common symptom for patients with MS. Treatment normally involves timed voiding, fluid restriction, and anticholinergic or antimuscarinic drugs, as long as postvoid residual urine volumes are less than 100 mL. Typically extended-release oxybutynin or tolterodine are first-line treatments. Botulinum toxin injection is considered for patients resistant to treatment. Some patients will require intermittent catheterizations or in-dwelling catheter. [163]

Sexual dysfunction also is common in about 50% of patients, and treatment is the same as for the general population.[163] There is a higher incidence of seizures for patients with MS; patients tend to respond well to antiepileptic drugs, if needed.[176] Dementia is uncommon for patients with MS (about 5%), but mild cognitive dysfunction is common (up to 70%).[177] The benefit of cholinesterase inhibitors for patients with MS is unclear at this time.[163] Gait impairment also is a very common symptom; some studies have shown modest benefit with dalfampridine (4-aminopyridine), which should be considered.[178]

### Amyotrophic Lateral Sclerosis

The management of ALS is based on symptoms. Riluzole, a glutamate antagonist, is the only FDA-approved drug for ALS, and studies demonstrate that riluzole slows the progression of ALS and prolongs survival by 83 days (median).[179-181] The use of noninvasive positive-pressure ventilation (NPPV) with bilevel positive airway pressure (BiPAP) also has demonstrated survival benefit and improved QOL.[182] Criteria for the use of NPPV are vital capacity less than 50% of predicted, presence of orthopnea, sniff nasal inspiratory force less than 40 cm, maximal inspiratory pressure less than 60 cm, or nocturnal oximetry less than 88%.[183]

Invasive ventilation or diaphragmatic pacing also can be considered. Dysphagia is common for patients with ALS, and limited data suggest that percutaneous gastrostomy (PEG) tube placement is associated with prolonged survival, although the degree of survival advantage is uncertain.[182,183] Typically this is considered for patients with 10% weight loss, those who require 30 minutes or more to finish their meals, or for patients with symptomatic dysphagia (coughing/choking). Sialorrhea (drooling) is a common complaint and can be treated with atropine, hyoscyamine, amitriptyline, glycopyrrolate, botulinum toxin injection (into parotid or submandibular gland), or low-dose radiation to the salivary gland. Mucolytic enzymes can be considered if the mucus is thick. Pseudobulbar affect is common as ALS progresses, and treatment options include dextromethorphan-quinidine, tricyclic antidepressants (eg, amitriptyline), or SSRIs (eg, fluvoxamine).[182,184] A common side effect of riluzole is fatigue; a trial with a stimulant such as modafinil may be helpful.[185] ALS-associated spasticity can be treated with a trial of either baclofen or tizanidine.[186] Pain, depression, and sleep disorders also are common, and the first step in management is to identify and treat any underlying causes. If none are found, then symptomatic treatment should be considered. The short survival rate and high symptom burden for patients with ALS necessitates a multidisciplinary approach, and these patients receive substantial benefit from palliative and hospice care.

## Clinical Situation

### Frank

Frank is a 69-year-old man who is experiencing a 1-month history of weakness in his left foot. Upon further questioning, he also reports right arm weakness and muscle cramps in his legs. He reports no additional symptoms. Frank denies any bladder or bowel dysfunction. He is otherwise healthy and takes no medications. On exam you notice he has some atrophy of his proximal muscles of his right arm and distal muscle weakness with fasciculations. He also has some tongue fasciculations. Deep tendon reflexes are brisk, and he has a bilateral extensor plantar response. He experiences no sensory loss, and his lab work is within normal limits.

 What is the most likely diagnosis?

This patient most likely has ALS. Patients with ALS typically have asymmetric progressive painless weakness (extremities or bulbar) on presentation. Also, the lack of bowel and bladder problems and sensory loss that would indicate cervical myelopathy and the combination of upper motor neuron findings (hyperreflexia, extensor plantar response) and lower motor neurons (atrophy, fasciculations) strongly suggest ALS. The combination of upper motor neuron findings (hyperreflexia, extensor plantar response) and lower motor neuron signs (atrophy, fasciculations) strongly suggests ALS. Patients with copper deficiency myeloneuropathy typically present with abnormal gait, sensory impairment (impaired vibration/proprioception), and spasticity. Guillain-Barre Syndrome's classical features are progressive symmetrical muscle weakness (normally starting in the legs) with absent/depressed deep tendon reflexes for days/weeks, which aren't Frank's symptoms.

Which treatment(s) have been shown to increase survival in patients with ALS?

Riluzole has been shown to slow the progression of ALS and prolong survival by a median of 83 days. The use of NPPV with BiPAP also has shown survival benefit and improved QOL. Limited data suggest that PEG-tube placement is associated with prolonged survival, although the degree of survival advantage is uncertain. There are no randomized controlled trials to indicate whether enteral-tube feeding is beneficial compared with continuation of oral feeding for any of the outcome measures for ALS patients. The best evidence suggests a survival advantage for some people with ALS/motor neuron disease, but these conclusions are tentative. Evidence for improved nutrition is also incomplete but tentatively favorable. QOL has been addressed in a few studies, but further studies are needed. In nonrandomized studies comparing surgical and radiographic approaches to feeding tube insertion, these two procedures for PEG tube insertion appear to be equivalent.[187]

 What factors portend a better prognosis in ALS?

Younger age appears to be a better prognostic factor. The main risk factors for ALS are age and family history. There are no conclusive data that suggest gender plays a significant role. Additional factors thought to be associated with poor prognosis are bulbar or respiratory onset disease, frontotemporal dementia, forced vital capacity less than 50%, a short interval from first symptom to diagnosis, malnutrition (BMI less than 25), sniff nasal inspiratory pressure (less than 40 cm/$H_2O$), and a high level of psychological distress.[128-131]

## End-Stage Issues

The management of neurological conditions for patients at the end of life consists of management of underlying symptoms to optimize QOL, advance care planning, management of total pain, and, at times, withdrawal of nonbeneficial life-sustaining treatments. Because of the high symptom burden experienced by patients with neurological conditions, a multidisciplinary management approach is needed.

There are many challenges that occur in the management neurological diseases for patients at the end of life. These include a sometimes long duration of disease, sudden death, lack of predictable course or fluctuating course, complex multidisciplinary care, neuropsychiatric symptoms, and communication problems, along with the fact that neurological conditions are widely variable.

## Communication and Decision-Making Capacity

Because many patients with underlying neurological conditions will have communication difficulties at some point in their disease course (secondary to dysarthria, dementia, respiratory problems, or coma), early advance care planning is essential. At times when the course is sudden (eg, stroke), effective communication with families that is both empathetic and honest is needed.[12] Advance care planning should include discussing the typical disease course, estimated prognosis and prognostic limitations, treatment options, completion of advance directives, and goals of care. Also, because dysphagia is common in patients with underlying neurological conditions, consideration of artificial nutrition and hydration is important early in the disease course. The loss of communication can have a large psychological impact on patients and family members, often requiring the involvement of a psychologist, speech-language pathologist, and occupational therapist, along with pastoral care and a social worker to help patients and families adjust. There also are multiple technologies available for patients that can help resolve communication barriers, such as smartphones, speech generating devices, and electronic eye gaze. The use of these augmentative/alternative communication devices also will help determine if a patient has decision-making capacity, which can be challenging with patients who have severe communication impairments.[188] See *UNIPAC 5* for more information about communicating with patients and families and decision making. See *UNIPAC 6* for more information about advance care planning and decision-making capacity.

## Dysphagia and Nutrition

Patients with chronic neurological diseases are at high risk of developing malnutrition, typically secondary to dysphagia. Up to 50% of patients with stroke will develop dysphagia, typically oropharyngeal in nature.[189] Thus, it is important to assess swallowing function in every patient after stroke, especially as dysphagia is associated with a three-fold increase in mortality and six-fold increase in aspiration.[189] Most patients will recover their swallowing function after one month following a stroke. Treatments typically consist of rehabilitation, simple maneuvers (chin tuck), modified diet, and sometimes the use of a nasogastric (NG) or PEG tube.

Malnutrition also is common for patients with MS. There are many possible etiologies, including reduced mobility and fatigue (difficulty shopping and cooking), physical difficulties manipulating food and fluid into their mouth, impaired vision, decreased appetite, reduced cognition, dysphagia, and medication side effects. Dysphagia occurs in up to 30% of patients with MS.[190] Treatment is based on identifying the etiology and trying to intervene, if possible.[190] As stated above, dysphagia is common in ALS and may even be the presenting symptom for patients with bulbar ALS. Limited data suggest that PEG tubes may have a survival advantage for some people with ALS/motor neuron disease, but these conclusions are tentative.[183] For patients with a vital capacity less than 30%, PEG tube is normally not considered, but comfort feeding versus palliative hydration or NG-tube feeding can be considered.[183]

Malnutrition and dysphagia occur in up to 95% of patients in the late stages of PD.[191] PD is associated with oropharyngeal dysphagia, gastroparesis, and constipation. When dysphagia is present, the mean survival is about 2 years, and patients typically are entering the palliative phase of their disease.[191] Titrating medications to increase the "on" motor stages can help. This can be accomplished by orally disintegrating carbidopa-levodopa (Parcopa), a rotigotine patch, subcutaneous apomorphine, or duodenal infusion of levodopa (Duodopa). Each of these therapies is expensive, and the value of each therapy in the context of QOL and cost must be weighed carefully, particularly as patients transition to hospice. The placement of deep brain neurostimulators also may help improve motor function. Dietary changes such as modified food, specialized utensils, rehabilitation, simple maneuvers (chin tuck), and low-protein diets may help. It is theorized that amino acids compete with levodopa for transportation across the blood-brain barrier, and it is postulated that low-protein diets may improve drug uptake and enhance mobility, although further research is needed.[192] There is no conclusive evidence that PEG-tube placement will increase survival in patients with PD, and pneumonia, typically aspiration pneumonia, continues to be a leading cause of death for patients with PD. The general recommendations are that PEG tubes should only be used in four conditions: head and neck cancer, acute stroke with dysphagia, ALS, and gastric decompression.[193] Thus, early advance care planning regarding artificial nutrition and hydration is essential for patients with chronic neurological conditions.

### Withdrawing Nonbeneficial Life-Sustaining Treatment

For patients with underlying neurological conditions who require life-sustaining treatments, the decision to withdrawal life supports associated with more burden than benefit can be extremely difficult for the patient (if able to participate) and family members. As part of advance care planning, clinicians should discuss a range of treatment options within the context of a progressive neurologic illness, including the role of time-limited trials. It also is important to discuss with patients and family members their preference regarding organ donation before withdrawal. When the decision is made to withdraw life-sustaining therapies, it is very important for providers to be prepared to manage any symptom that the patient may experience. This typically includes dyspnea, pain, and anxiety/agitation. It also is important to communicate with patients and families that death is imminent.[12,144] Providers should counsel family members about anticipated signs and symptoms of the dying process after treatment withdrawals and prepare family members that death may or may not occur shortly after discontinuation. Many hospitals and hospices have protocols for withdrawal of life-sustaining treatments to ensure optimal symptom management and adherence to patient goals.[12] Medications at bedside should consist of opioids for pain and dyspnea, anticholinergics for increased secretions (although no large-scale study has confirmed their efficacy), anxiolytics and other sedatives to help with agitation/anxiety, and potentially antiepileptic medications in the event of a seizure.[12] It also is important to discontinue any therapies and medications that are not contributing to the comfort of the patient. Palliative sedation may be considered for patients who have a terminal illness and experience uncontrolled symptoms (eg, pain, dyspnea, delirium, convulsions). In small studies, palliative sedation does not appear to hasten death.[194] Family support during this withdrawal process is crucial, along with bereavement counseling to help with the grief over the loss of the loved one.

## Palliative Care and Hospice

The course of neurological conditions is highly variable, and prognosis can be challenging at the time of diagnosis. Most treatments for neurological conditions are palliative in nature because these diseases are largely incurable. They also have a high symptom burden, and studies demonstrate that the burden can equal that of metastatic cancer.[1,195] The protracted course and accumulating disability leads to caregiver burden that is similar to that of caregivers of patients with cancer.[196] The high rates of physical, psychological, and cognitive disabilities among patients with neurologic illnesses create a very conducive model for incorporating palliative care principles early in the disease course.[1] Patients with neurological conditions especially suffer from high rates of demoralization, hopelessness, depression, and even suicide, which appear higher than in patients with metastatic cancer.[197] Although palliative care in general is shown to improve patient satisfaction, achieve higher QOL, prolong life, and decrease cost, studies specific to neurological conditions generally are lacking.[198-200] See *UNIPAC 2* for information on assessing and treating psychiatric and psychological conditions related to serious illness.

In the United States, the Medicare hospice benefit is available when the medical prognosis is 6 months or less if the disease runs its expected course and the patient has chosen—directly or through a surrogate—to focus on comfort. **Table 27** lists hospice eligibility guidelines for specific neurologic conditions. The National Hospice and Palliative Care Organization estimated that in 2014 approximately 44.6% of all deaths in the United States were of patients receiving hospice care, although hospice utilization is low among patients with underlying neurological conditions.[201] It also was estimated that in 2014, 6.4% of hospice admissions were from stroke or coma patients, 0.4% from patients with ALS, and 2.1% from patients with other neurological conditions (excluding dementia). Median length of stay on hospice was low, estimated in 2014 to be about 17 days, with 35% having a length of stay less than 7 days.[201] For patients not receiving hospice, in-hospital death rates were considerably higher than for patients receiving hospice for PD (45% vs 0.6%) and MS (56% vs 2.5%).[202] There are many potential barriers to hospice referrals, including fear of taking hope away from patients and family members, limited training of physicians in primary palliative care, inadequate number of palliative care physicians, and conservative and nonspecific Medicare hospice guidelines for neurological conditions. Disease progression associated with a prognosis of 6 months or less includes ADL dependence, multiple hospitalizations, unexplained weight loss, dysphagia, and rapid decline in function.[1] Most patients with ALS will die as a result of respiratory failure.[203] Early stroke mortality is secondary to neurological complications, while later mortality appears secondary to respiratory and cardiovascular causes.[204] In patients with PD, mortality typically is secondary to respiratory infection, dementia, cardiovascular disease or fracture. The cause of mortality in patients with MS typically is secondary to cardiovascular disease (eg, acute myocardial infarction, cardiovascular accident), infection, suicide, and cancer, with infection being the leading cause.[205] Studies examining the benefit of palliative care and hospice in advanced neurologic illness represent a ripe area for further inquiry. See *UNIPAC 1* for more information on hospice care.

## Table 27. CMS Hospice Guidelines for Neurological Disorders[206]

| | |
|---|---|
| **Stroke** | KPS or PPS score of 40% or less and inability to maintain hydration and caloric intake with one of the following:<br>• weight loss of more than 10% in the last 6 months or more than 7.5% in the last 3 months<br>• serum albumin of less than 2.5 g/dL<br>• current history of pulmonary aspiration not responsive to speech-language pathology intervention<br>• sequential calorie counts documenting inadequate caloric/fluid intake<br>• dysphagia severe enough to prevent the patient from receiving food and fluids necessary to sustain life, in a patient who declines or does not receive artificial nutrition and hydration. |
| **Coma** | Comatose patients with any three of the following on day 3 of coma:<br>• abnormal brain stem response<br>• absent verbal response<br>• absent withdrawal response to pain<br>• serum creatinine greater than 1.5 mg/dL.<br>Documentation of medical complications, in the context of progressive clinical decline, within the previous 12 months, which support a terminal prognosis:<br>• aspiration pneumonia<br>• upper urinary tract infection (pyelonephritis)<br>• sepsis<br>• refractory stage 3-4 decubitus ulcers<br>• fever recurrent after antibiotics.<br>Documentation of diagnostic imaging factors that support poor prognosis after stroke include<br>• for nontraumatic hemorrhagic stroke<br>  » large-volume hemorrhage on CT: infratentorial: ≥ 20 mL; supratentorial: ≥ 50 mL<br>  » ventricular extension of hemorrhage<br>  » surface area of involvement of hemorrhage ≥ 30% of cerebrum<br>  » midline shift ≥ 1.5 cm<br>  » obstructive hydrocephalus in patient who declines, or is not a candidate for, ventriculoperitoneal shunt<br>• for thrombotic/embolic stroke<br>  » large anterior infarcts with both cortical and subcortical involvement<br>  » large bihemispheric infarcts<br>  » basilar artery occlusion<br>  » bilateral vertebral artery occlusion. |

*Continued on page 143*

## Table 27. CMS Hospice Guidelines for Neurological Disorders[206] *(continued)*

| | |
|---|---|
| **ALS** | Critically impaired breathing capacity as demonstrated by all the following characteristics occurring within the 12 months preceding initial hospice certification: |

**ALS**      Critically impaired breathing capacity as demonstrated by all the following characteristics occurring within the 12 months preceding initial hospice certification:

- vital capacity less than 30% of normal (if available)
- dyspnea at rest
- patient declines mechanical ventilation; external ventilation used for comfort measures only.

Rapid progression of ALS or neurological condition as demonstrated by all the following characteristics occurring within the 12 months preceding initial hospice certification:

- progression from independent ambulation to wheelchair to bed-bound status
- progression from normal to barely intelligible or unintelligible speech
- progression from normal to pureed diet
- progression from independence in most or all ADLs to needing major assistance by caretaker in all ADLs.

Critical nutritional impairment as demonstrated by all the following characteristics occurring within the 12 months preceding initial hospice certification:

- oral intake of nutrients and fluids insufficient to sustain life
- continuing weight loss
- dehydration or hypovolemia
- absence of artificial feeding methods sufficient to sustain life but not for relieving hunger.

Life-threatening complications as demonstrated by one of the following characteristics occurring within the 12 months preceding initial hospice certification:

- recurrent aspiration pneumonia (with or without tube feedings)
- upper urinary tract infection, eg, pyelonephritis
- sepsis
- recurrent fever after antibiotic therapy
- stage 3 or 4 decubitus ulcer(s).

*Continued on page 144*

## Table 27. CMS Hospice Guidelines for Neurological Disorders[206] (continued)

| | |
|---|---|
| **Generic criteria for other neurologic illnesses, including PD, MS, MD, or MG** | Terminal condition<br>Rapid decline over the past 3-6 months as evidenced by progression of disease by clinical status, symptoms, signs and labs<br>Physiologic impairment of functional status as demonstrated by KPS or PPS of less than 70%. Note that three of the disease specific guidelines (HIV, stroke, and coma) establish a lower qualifying KPS or PPS.<br>Dependence on assistance for two or more ADLs:<br>• feeding<br>• ambulation<br>• continence<br>• transfer<br>• bathing<br>• dressing.<br>Increasing emergency room visits, hospitalizations, or physician's visits related to hospice primary diagnosis<br>Progressive stage 3-4 pressure ulcer(s) in spite of optimal care. |

*ADLs, activities of daily living; ALS, amytrophic lateral sclerosis; CT, computed tomography; HIV, human immunodeficiency virus; KPS, Karnofsky Performance Status; MD, muscular dystrophy; MG, myasthenia gravis; MS, multiple sclerosis; PD, Parkinson's disease; PPS, Palliative Performance Scale*

*Note. See local coverage determinations (LCDs) for specifics.[206] LCDs vary by Medicare Administrative Contractor (MAC). Use the specific LCDs provided by your region's MAC when documenting hospice eligibility.*

## Issues for Caregivers

Patients with neurological conditions experience loss of function, communication problems, dysphagia, cognitive impairments, and high rates of psychological and other symptoms over their disease course. For this reason, family members and other caregivers often play a vital role in their lives. These conditions also are extremely difficult for loved ones and caregivers because the burden of these diseases can occur over many years. These diseases not only affect a patient's ability to function, they can also affect a patient's personality and cognitive ability. The emotional impact of watching a loved one's decline over many years can take a huge toll.

Almost 90% of caregivers are unpaid and more than 80% are women. Multiple studies have shown high rates of stress, burnout, depression, impaired QOL, and overall poor health among caregivers of patients with chronic neurological conditions.[207-210] Caregiver burden appears to be greater when patients have cognitive and behavioral problems, bladder dysfunction, and more restrictions in their ADLs.[209,211] There also appears to be a strong association between a caregiver's mental health status and caregiver burden.[209] Additional risk factors associated with adverse outcomes among caregivers appear to be advanced age, high dependency, female sex, low educational attainment, shared residence with the care recipient, higher number of hours spent caregiving, depression, social isolation, financial stress, lack of choice in being a caregiver, and poor family support.[212,213] One study showed that anxiety was present in 17% of caregivers compared with 10% in a control group.[214] Another landmark study showed that caregiver strain was associated with 63% higher mortality than for noncaregiver controls.[215] Additional studies have shown high rates of weight loss, low self-esteem, depression, social isolation, suicide, and financial stress for caregivers.[215,216] Thus, it is very important to screen for caregiver stress and burden. Many assessment tools are available, including the Zarit Burden Interview, Caregiver Assessment Tool, Caregiver Reaction Scale, Caregiver Burden Scale, Caregiver Strain Index, and Screen for Caregiver Burden. Of these scales, the Zarit Burden Interview is the most widely used.[217]

There are psychosocial and psychological interventions that appear to have some efficacy at mitigating caregiver burden. These include neurological-disease-specific support groups, psychoeducational interventions for caregivers, respite, antidepressants, and management of patients' underlying behavioral problems.[213] Respite care services are available in the community at diverse sites as well as through hospice. This can help relieve the caregiver from the day-to-day burden of caring for the patient. Adult day care services can be an excellent source of respite for caregivers. It also is important to screen for elder abuse because rates are higher among caregivers with high burden. It is important to engage case managers and social workers to help obtain additional resources, if possible, and to help patients and families navigate the healthcare system and manage stressors. Bereavement support will be critical because a caregiver's identify often is tied to their loved one, and grief about the loss of their loved one can be very difficult. The following resources are helpful for patients and families who are seeking information about the support groups that are available (All accessible as of August 4, 2017):

- National Multiple Sclerosis Society—www.nationalmssociety.org/Resources-Support/Find-Support/Join-a-Local-Support-Group
- ALS Association—www.alsa.org/community/support-groups/
- American Heart Association/American Stroke Association—www.strokeassociation.org/STROKEORG/strokegroup/public/zipFinder.jsp
- National Parkinson Foundation—www.parkinson.org/find-help/resources-in-your-community
- Huntington's Disease Society of America—hdsa.org/about-hdsa/support-groups.
  See *UNIPAC 2* for more information about caregiving.

# References

1. Boersma I, Miyasaki J, Kutner J, Kluger B. Palliative care and neurology: time for a paradigm shift. *Neurology.* 2014;83(6):561-567.

2. Dallara A, Tolchin DW. Emerging subspecialties in neurology: palliative care. *Neurology.* 2014;82(7):640-642.

3. Hussain J, Adams D, Campbell C. End-of-life care in neurodegenerative conditions: outcomes of a specialist palliative neurology service. *Int J Palliat Nurs.* 2013;19(4):162-169.

4. Turner-Stokes L, Sykes N, Silber E, Khatri A, Sutton L, Young E. From diagnosis to death: exploring the interface between neurology, rehabilitation and palliative care in managing people with long-term neurological conditions. *Clin Med (Lond).* 2007;7(2):129-136.

5. Turner-Stokes L, Sykes N, Silber E, Guideline Development G. Long-term neurological conditions: management at the interface between neurology, rehabilitation and palliative care. *Clin Med (Lond).* 2008;8(2):186-191.

6. Dallara A, Meret A, Saroyan J. Mapping the literature: palliative care within adult and child neurology. *J Child Neurol.* 2014;29(12):1728-1738.

7. Borasio GD, Voltz R. [Patient consultation and palliative care in neurology, e.g. in amyotrophic lateral sclerosis]. *Internist (Berl).* 2000;41(7):627-632.

8. Koekkoek JA, Chang S, Taphoorn MJ. Palliative care at the end-of-life in glioma patients. *Handb Clin Neurol.* 2016;134:315-326.

9. Karam CY, Paganoni S, Joyce N, Carter GT, Bedlack R. Palliative care issues in amyotrophic lateral sclerosis: An evidenced-based review. *Am J Hosp Palliat Care.* 2016;33(1):84-92.

10. Eriksson H, Milberg A, Hjelm K, Friedrichsen M. End of life care for patients dying of stroke: a comparative registry study of stroke and cancer. *PLoS One.* 2016;11(2):e0147694.

11. Miyasaki JM, Kluger B. Palliative care for Parkinson's disease: has the time come? *Curr Neurol Neurosci Rep.* 2015;15(5):26.

12. Frontera JA, Curtis JR, Nelson JE, et al. Integrating palliative care into the care of neurocritically ill patients: a report from the Improving Palliative Care in the ICU Project Advisory Board and the Center to Advance Palliative Care. *Crit Care Med.* 2015;43(9):1964-1977.

13. Borasio GD. The role of palliative care in patients with neurological diseases. *Nat Rev Neurol.* 2013;9(5):292-295.

14. Palliative care in neurology. The American Academy of Neurology Ethics and Humanities Subcommittee. *Neurology.* 1996;46(3):870-872.

15. Accreditation Council for Graduate Medical Education. ACGME Program Requirements for Graduate Medical Education in Neurology. www.acgme.org/Portals/0/PFAssets/ProgramRequirements/180_neurology_2016.pdf?ver=2016-09-30-123013-030. Accessed June 30, 2017.

16. Gilman S, Wenning GK, Low PA, et al. Second consensus statement on the diagnosis of multiple system atrophy. *Neurology.* 2008;71(9):670-676.

17. Creutzfeldt CJ, Robinson MT, Holloway RG. Neurologists as primary palliative care providers: communication and practice approaches. *Neurol Clin Pract.* 2016;6(1):40-48.

18. National Center for Health Statistics, Centers for Disease Control and Prevention, US Department of Health and Human Services. Cerebrovascular disease or stroke. www.cdc.gov/nchs/fastats/stroke.htm. Accessed June 29, 2017.

19. Feigin VL, Lawes CM, Bennett DA, Anderson CS. Stroke epidemiology: a review of population-based studies of incidence, prevalence, and case-fatality in the late 20th century. *Lancet Neurol.* 2003;2(1):43-53.

20. American College of Physicians. *MKSAP 16: Neurology.* Philadelphia, PA: American College of Physicians; 2012.

21. Stevens T, Payne SA, Burton C, Addington-Hall J, Jones A. Palliative care in stroke: a critical review of the literature. *Palliat Med*. 2007;21(4):323-331.

22. van der Worp HB, van Gijn J. Acute Ischemic Stroke. *N Engl J Med*. 2007;357(6):572-579.

23. Caplan L. Overview of the evaluation of stroke. *UpToDate*. https://www.uptodate.com/contents/overview-of-the-evaluation-of-stroke. Accessed June 30, 2017.

24. Dawson J, Walters M. Development and validation of a stroke recognition tool. *Lancet Neurol*. 2005;4(11):691-693.

25. Olanow C, Schapira A, Obeso J. Parkinson's Disease and Other Movement Disorders. In: Kasper D, Fauci A, Hauser S, Longo D, Jameson J, Loscalzo J, eds. *Harrison's Principles of Internal Medicine*. 19 ed. New York, NY: McGraw-Hill; 2015.

26. Jankovic J, Fahn S. Physiologic and pathologic tremors. Diagnosis, mechanism, and management. *Ann Intern Med*. 1980;93(3):460-465.

27. Albanese A, Bhatia K, Bressman SB, et al. Phenomenology and classification of dystonia: a consensus update. *Mov Disord*. 2013;28(7):863-873.

28. Bhidayasiri R, Truong DD. Chorea and related disorders. *Postgrad Med J*. 2004;80(947):527-534.

29. Timmann D, Diener H. Coordination and Ataxia. In: Goetz CG, ed. *Textbook of Clinical Neurology*. 3 ed. Philadelphia, PA: Saunders; 2007:307.

30. Marsden C, Hallett M, Fahn S. In: Fahn S, ed. *Movement Disorders*. London, UK: Butterworths; 1982:196.

31. Zupancic M, Mahajan A, Handa K. Dementia with lewy bodies: diagnosis and management for primary care providers. *Prim Care Companion CNS Disord*. 2011;13(5).

32. Zielonka D, Mielcarek M, Landwehrmeyer GB. Update on Huntington's disease: advances in care and emerging therapeutic options. *Parkinsonism Relat Disord*. 2015;21(3):169-178.

33. Litvan I, Mangone CA, McKee A, et al. Natural history of progressive supranuclear palsy (Steele-Richardson-Olszewski syndrome) and clinical predictors of survival: a clinicopathological study. *J Neurol Neurosurg Psychiatry*. 1996;60(6):615-620.

34. Respondek G, Roeber S, Kretzschmar H, et al. Accuracy of the National Institute for Neurological Disorders and Stroke/Society for Progressive Supranuclear Palsy and neuroprotection and natural history in Parkinson plus syndromes criteria for the diagnosis of progressive supranuclear palsy. *Mov Disord*. 2013;28(4):504-509.

35. Milligan SA, Chesson AL. Restless legs syndrome in the older adult: diagnosis and management. *Drugs Aging*. 2002;19(10):741-751.

36. Czeisler C, Scammell T, Saper C. Sleep Disorders. In: Kasper D, Fauci A, Hauser S, Longo D, Jameson J, Loscalzo J, eds. *Harrison's Principles of Internal Medicine*. 19 ed. New York, NY: McGraw-Hill; 2015.

37. Dawson S, Kristjanson LJ, Toye CM, Flett P. Living with Huntington's disease: need for supportive care. *Nurs Health Sci*. 2004;6(2):123-130.

38. Marks S, Hung S, Rosielle DA. Palliative care for patients with Huntington's disease #201. *J Palliat Med*. 2011;14(5):655-656.

39. Postuma RB, Berg D, Stern M, et al. MDS clinical diagnostic criteria for Parkinson's disease. *Mov Disord*. 2015;30(12):1591-1601.

40. Seifert KD, Wiener JI. The impact of DaTscan on the diagnosis and management of movement disorders: A retrospective study. *Am J Neurodegener Dis*. 2013;2(1):29-34.

41. Goetz CG, Tilley BC, Shaftman SR, et al. Movement Disorder Society-sponsored revision of the Unified Parkinson's Disease Rating Scale (MDS-UPDRS): scale presentation and clinimetric testing results. *Mov Disord*. 2008;23(15):2129-2170.

42. Hauser S, Goodin D. Multiple Sclerosis and Other Demyelinating Diseases. In: Kasper D, Fauci A, Hauser S, Longo D, Jameson J, Loscalzo J, eds. *Harrison's Principles of Internal Medicine*. 19 ed. New York, NY: McGraw-Hill; 2015.

43. Polman CH, Reingold SC, Banwell B, et al. Diagnostic criteria for multiple sclerosis: 2010 revisions to the McDonald criteria. *Ann Neurol*. 2011;69(2):292-302.

44. Filippi M, Rocca MA. MR imaging of multiple sclerosis. *Radiology*. 2011;259(3):659-681.

45. Brooks BR. El Escorial World Federation of Neurology criteria for the diagnosis of amyotrophic lateral sclerosis. Subcommittee on Motor Neuron Diseases/Amyotrophic Lateral Sclerosis of the World Federation of Neurology Research Group on Neuromuscular Diseases and the El Escorial "Clinical limits of amyotrophic lateral sclerosis" workshop contributors. *J Neurol Sci*. 1994;124 Suppl:96-107.

46. Brooks BR, Miller RG, Swash M, Munsat TL. El Escorial revisited: revised criteria for the diagnosis of amyotrophic lateral sclerosis. *Amyotroph Lateral Scler Other Motor Neuron Disord*. 2000;1(5):293-299.

47. Hemphill JC, 3rd, Bonovich DC, Besmertis L, Manley GT, Johnston SC. The ICH score: a simple, reliable grading scale for intracerebral hemorrhage. *Stroke*. 2001;32(4):891-897.

48. Rost NS, Smith EE, Chang Y, et al. Prediction of functional outcome in patients with primary intracerebral hemorrhage: the FUNC score. *Stroke*. 2008;39(8):2304-2309.

49. van Asch CJ, Luitse MJ, Rinkel GJ, van der Tweel I, Algra A, Klijn CJ. Incidence, case fatality, and functional outcome of intracerebral haemorrhage over time, according to age, sex, and ethnic origin: a systematic review and meta-analysis. *Lancet Neurol*. 2010;9(2):167-176.

50. Rodriguez-Luna D, Rubiera M, Ribo M, et al. Serum low-density lipoprotein cholesterol level predicts hematoma growth and clinical outcome after acute intracerebral hemorrhage. *Stroke*. 2011;42(9):2447-2452.

51. Hackam DG, Woodward M, Newby LK, et al. Statins and intracerebral hemorrhage: collaborative systematic review and meta-analysis. *Circulation*. 2011;124(20):2233-2242.

52. Mozaffarian D, Benjamin E, Go A, et al. Heart disease and stroke statistics—2016 update: a report from the American Heart Association. *Circulation*. 2016;133(4):e38-360.

53. Go AS, Mozaffarian D, Roger VL, et al. Heart Disease and Stroke Statistics—2014 Update: A Report From the American Heart Association. *Circulation*. 2014;129(3):e28-e292.

54. Saposnik G, Kapral MK, Liu Y, et al. IScore: a risk score to predict death early after hospitalization for an acute ischemic stroke. *Circulation*. 2011;123(7):739-749.

55. Aminoff M, Greenberg D, Simon R. Stroke. In: Aminoff M, Greenberg D, Simon R, eds. *Clinical Neurology*. 9 ed. New York, NY: McGraw-Hill; 2015.

56. Pringsheim T, Jette N, Frolkis A, Steeves TD. The prevalence of Parkinson's disease: a systematic review and meta-analysis. *Mov Disord*. 2014;29(13):1583-1590.

57. Jankovic J. Etiology and pathogenesis of Parkinson disease. *UpToDate*. https://www.uptodate.com/contents/etiology-and-pathogenesis-of-parkinson-disease. Accessed June 30, 2017.

58. de Lau LM, Breteler MM. Epidemiology of Parkinson's disease. *Lancet Neurol*. 2006;5(6):525-535.

59. Kingsbury AE, Bandopadhyay R, Silveira-Moriyama L, et al. Brain stem pathology in Parkinson's disease: an evaluation of the Braak staging model. *Mov Disord*. 2010;25(15):2508-2515.

60. Noyce AJ, Bestwick JP, Silveira-Moriyama L, et al. Meta-analysis of early nonmotor features and risk factors for Parkinson disease. *Ann Neurol*. 2012;72(6):893-901.

61. Kieburtz K, Wunderle KB. Parkinson's disease: evidence for environmental risk factors. *Mov Disord*. 2013;28(1):8-13.

62. Hedstrom AK, Alfredsson L, Olsson T. Environmental factors and their interactions with risk genotypes in MS susceptibility. *Curr Opin Neurol*. 2016;29(3):293-298.

63. Ascherio A, Munger KL. Environmental risk factors for multiple sclerosis. Part II: Noninfectious factors. *Ann Neurol.* 2007;61(6):504-513.

64. Ascherio A, Munger KL. Environmental risk factors for multiple sclerosis. Part I: the role of infection. *Ann Neurol.* 2007;61(4):288-299.

65. Ascherio A, Munger K. Epidemiology of multiple sclerosis: from risk factors to prevention. *Semin Neurol.* 2008;28(1):17-28.

66. National Multiple Sclerosis Society. Epidemiology and Causation. www.nationalmssociety.org/For-Professionals/Clinical-Care/About-MS/Epidemiology-and-Causation. Accessed June 30, 2017.

67. Adelman G, Rane SG, Villa KF. The cost burden of multiple sclerosis in the United States: a systematic review of the literature. *J Med Econ.* 2013;16(5):639-647.

68. Lublin FD, Reingold SC, Cohen JA, et al. Defining the clinical course of multiple sclerosis: the 2013 revisions. *Neurology.* 2014;83(3):278-286.

69. Worms PM. The epidemiology of motor neuron diseases: a review of recent studies. *J Neurol Sci.* 2001;191(1-2):3-9.

70. Logroscino G, Traynor BJ, Hardiman O, et al. Incidence of amyotrophic lateral sclerosis in Europe. *J Neurol Neurosurg Psychiatry.* 2010;81(4):385-390.

71. Jordan H, Rechtman L, Wagner L, Kaye WE. Amyotrophic lateral sclerosis surveillance in Baltimore and Philadelphia. *Muscle Nerve.* 2015;51(6):815-821.

72. Peters OM, Ghasemi M, Brown RH, Jr. Emerging mechanisms of molecular pathology in ALS. *J Clin Invest.* 2015;125(5):1767-1779.

73. Su FC, Goutman SA, Chernyak S, et al. Association of environmental toxins with amyotrophic lateral sclerosis. *JAMA Neurol.* 2016;73(7):803-811.

74. Kurland LT, Mulder DW. Epidemiologic investigations of amyotrophic lateral sclerosis. I. Preliminary report on geographic distribution, with special reference to the Mariana Islands, including clinical and pathologic observations. *Neurology.* 1954;4(5):355-378.

75. Weisskopf MG, Cudkowicz ME, Johnson N. Military service and amyotrophic lateral sclerosis in a population-based cohort. *Epidemiology.* 2015;26(6):831-838.

76. Lomen-Hoerth C, Murphy J, Langmore S, Kramer JH, Olney RK, Miller B. Are amyotrophic lateral sclerosis patients cognitively normal? *Neurology.* 2003;60(7):1094-1097.

77. Esper CD, Factor SA. Failure of recognition of drug-induced parkinsonism in the elderly. *Mov Disord.* 2008;23(3):401-404.

78. Yashin A, Akushevich I, Ukraintseva S, Akushevich L, Arbeev K, Kulminski A. Trends in survival and recovery from stroke: evidence from the National Long-Term Care Survey/Medicare data. *Stroke.* 2010;41(3):563-565.

79. Theofanidis D, Fitsioris X, Iakovos T. Stroke scales and trajectory of recovery: a major concern for patients and nurses alike. *Health Science Journal.* 2015;9(4):1-7.

80. Kelly-Hayes M, Beiser A, Kase CS, Scaramucci A, D'Agostino RB, Wolf PA. The influence of gender and age on disability following ischemic stroke: the Framingham study. *J Stroke Cerebrovasc Dis.* 2003;12(3):119-126.

81. Dhamoon MS, Moon YP, Paik MC, Sacco RL, Elkind MS. Trajectory of functional decline before and after ischemic stroke: the Northern Manhattan Study. *Stroke.* 2012;43(8):2180-2184.

82. Casper M, Barnett E, Williams GJ, Halverson J, Braham V, Greenlund K. *Atlas of Stroke Mortality: Racial, Ethnic, and Geographic Disparities in the United States.* Atlanta, GA: Centers for Disease Control and Prevention, US Department of Health and Human Services; 2003.

83. Grysiewicz RA, Thomas K, Pandey DK. Epidemiology of ischemic and hemorrhagic stroke: incidence, prevalence, mortality, and risk factors. *Neurol Clin.* 2008;26(4):871-895, vii.

84. Edwardson M, Dromerick AW. Ischemic stroke prognosis in adults. *UpToDate*. https://www.uptodate.com/contents/ischemic-stroke-prognosis-in-adults. Accessed June 30, 2017.

85. Gonzalez-Perez A, Gaist D, Wallander MA, McFeat G, Garcia-Rodriguez LA. Mortality after hemorrhagic stroke: data from general practice (The Health Improvement Network). *Neurology*. 2013;81(6):559-565.

86. Smith EE, Shobha N, Dai D, et al. Risk score for in-hospital ischemic stroke mortality derived and validated within the Get With the Guidelines-Stroke Program. *Circulation*. 2010;122(15):1496-1504.

87. Papavasileiou V, Milionis H, Michel P, et al. ASTRAL score predicts 5-year dependence and mortality in acute ischemic stroke. *Stroke*. 2013;44(6):1616-1620.

88. Strbian D, Meretoja A, Ahlhelm FJ, et al. Predicting outcome of IV thrombolysis-treated ischemic stroke patients: the DRAGON score. *Neurology*. 2012;78(6):427-432.

89. Saposnik G, Reeves MJ, Johnston SC, Bath PM, Ovbiagele B. Predicting clinical outcomes after thrombolysis using the iScore: results from the Virtual International Stroke Trials Archive. *Stroke*. 2013;44(10):2755-2759.

90. O'Donnell MJ, Fang J, D'Uva C, et al. The PLAN score: a bedside prediction rule for death and severe disability following acute ischemic stroke. *Arch Intern Med*. 2012;172(20):1548-1556.

91. Weimar C, Konig IR, Kraywinkel K, Ziegler A, Diener HC. Age and National Institutes of Health Stroke Scale Score within 6 hours after onset are accurate predictors of outcome after cerebral ischemia: development and external validation of prognostic models. *Stroke*. 2004;35(1):158-162.

92. Adams HP, Jr., Davis PH, Leira EC, et al. Baseline NIH Stroke Scale score strongly predicts outcome after stroke: A report of the Trial of Org 10172 in Acute Stroke Treatment (TOAST). *Neurology*. 1999;53(1):126-131.

93. Koennecke HC, Belz W, Berfelde D, et al. Factors influencing in-hospital mortality and morbidity in patients treated on a stroke unit. *Neurology*. 2011;77(10):965-972.

94. Hankey GJ, Spiesser J, Hakimi Z, Bego G, Carita P, Gabriel S. Rate, degree, and predictors of recovery from disability following ischemic stroke. *Neurology*. 2007;68(19):1583-1587.

95. Andersen KK, Andersen ZJ, Olsen TS. Predictors of early and late case-fatality in a nationwide Danish study of 26,818 patients with first-ever ischemic stroke. *Stroke*. 2011;42(10):2806-2812.

96. Vogt G, Laage R, Shuaib A, Schneider A. Initial lesion volume is an independent predictor of clinical stroke outcome at day 90: an analysis of the Virtual International Stroke Trials Archive (VISTA) database. *Stroke*. 2012;43(5):1266-1272.

97. Konig IR, Ziegler A, Bluhmki E, et al. Predicting long-term outcome after acute ischemic stroke: a simple index works in patients from controlled clinical trials. *Stroke*. 2008;39(6):1821-1826.

98. Greer DM, Wang HH, Robinson JD, Varelas PN, Henderson GV, Wijdicks EF. Variability of brain death policies in the United States. *JAMA Neurol*. 2016;73(2):213-218.

99. Langhorne P, Stott DJ, Robertson L, et al. Medical complications after stroke: a multicenter study. *Stroke*. 2000;31(6):1223-1229.

100. Ingeman A, Andersen G, Hundborg HH, Svendsen ML, Johnsen SP. In-hospital medical complications, length of stay, and mortality among stroke unit patients. *Stroke*. 2011;42(11):3214-3218.

101. Feng W, Hendry RM, Adams RJ. Risk of recurrent stroke, myocardial infarction, or death in hospitalized stroke patients. *Neurology*. 2010;74(7):588-593.

102. Dromerick AW, Edwards DF, Diringer MN. Sensitivity to changes in disability after stroke: a comparison of four scales useful in clinical trials. *J Rehabil Res Dev*. 2003;40(1):1-8.

103. Goy ER, Carter J, Ganzini L. Neurologic disease at the end of life: caregiver descriptions of Parkinson disease and amyotrophic lateral sclerosis. *J Palliat Med*. 2008;11(4):548-554.

104. Macleod AD, Taylor KS, Counsell CE. Mortality in Parkinson's disease: a systematic review and meta-analysis. *Mov Disord*. 2014;29(13):1615-1622.

105. Diem-Zangerl A, Seppi K, Wenning GK, et al. Mortality in Parkinson's disease: a 20-year follow-up study. *Mov Disord*. 2009;24(6):819-825.

106. Velseboer DC, de Bie RM, Wieske L, et al. Development and external validation of a prognostic model in newly diagnosed Parkinson disease. *Neurology*. 2016;86(11):986-993.

107. Ishihara LS, Cheesbrough A, Brayne C, Schrag A. Estimated life expectancy of Parkinson's patients compared with the UK population. *J Neurol Neurosurg Psychiatry*. 2007;78(12):1304-1309.

108. Goetz CG, Poewe W, Rascol O, et al. Movement Disorder Society Task Force report on the Hoehn and Yahr staging scale: status and recommendations The Movement Disorder Society Task Force on rating scales for Parkinson's disease. *Mov Disord*. 2004;19(9):1020-1028.

109. Lokk J, Delbari A. Clinical aspects of palliative care in advanced Parkinson's disease. *BMC Palliat Care*. 2012;11:20.

110. Miyasaki JM. Palliative care in Parkinson's disease. *Curr Neurol Neurosci Rep*. 2013;13(8):367.

111. MacMahon DG, Thomas S. Practical approach to quality of life in Parkinson's disease: the nurse's role. *J Neurol*. 1998;245 Suppl 1:S19-22.

112. Richfield EW, Jones EJ, Alty JE. Palliative care for Parkinson's disease: a summary of the evidence and future directions. *Palliat Med*. 2013;27(9):805-810.

113. Thomas S, MacMahon D. Parkinson's disease, palliative care and older people: Part 1. *Nurs Older People*. 2004;16(1):22-26.

114. Lim SY, Fox SH, Lang AE. Overview of the extranigral aspects of Parkinson disease. *Arch Neurol*. 2009;66(2):167-172.

115. Barone P, Antonini A, Colosimo C, et al. The PRIAMO study: A multicenter assessment of nonmotor symptoms and their impact on quality of life in Parkinson's disease. *Mov Disord*. 2009;24(11):1641-1649.

116. Hussl A, Seppi K, Poewe W. Nonmotor symptoms in Parkinson's disease. *Expert Rev Neurother*. 2013;13(6):581-583.

117. Cummings JL. Intellectual impairment in Parkinson's disease: clinical, pathologic, and biochemical correlates. *J Geriatr Psychiatry Neurol*. 1988;1(1):24-36.

118. Olek M. Clinical course and classification of multiple sclerosis. *UpToDate*. https://www.uptodate.com/contents/clinical-course-and-classification-of-multiple-sclerosis. Accessed June 30, 2017.

119. National Multiple Sclerosis Society. Types of MS. www.nationalmssociety.org/What-is-MS/Types-of-MS. Accessed June 29, 2017.

120. Weinshenker BG. Natural history of multiple sclerosis. *Ann Neurol*. 1994;36 Suppl:S6-11.

121. Eriksson M, Andersen O, Runmarker B. Long-term follow up of patients with clinically isolated syndromes, relapsing-remitting and secondary progressive multiple sclerosis. *Mult Scler*. 2003;9(3):260-274.

122. Strupp J, Voltz R, Golla H. Opening locked doors: Integrating a palliative care approach into the management of patients with severe multiple sclerosis. *Mult Scler*. 2016;22(1):13-18.

123. Scalfari A, Knappertz V, Cutter G, Goodin DS, Ashton R, Ebers GC. Mortality in patients with multiple sclerosis. *Neurology*. 2013;81(2):184-192.

124. Rolak LA. Multiple sclerosis: it's not the disease you thought it was. *Clin Med Res*. 2003;1(1):57-60.

125. Manouchehrinia A, Tanasescu R, Tench CR, Constantinescu CS. Mortality in multiple sclerosis: meta-analysis of standardised mortality ratios. *J Neurol Neurosurg Psychiatry*. 2016;87(3):324-331.

126. Sadovnick AD, Eisen K, Ebers GC, Paty DW. Cause of death in patients attending multiple sclerosis clinics. *Neurology*. 1991;41(8):1193-1196.

127. Brenner P, Burkill S, Jokinen J, Hillert J, Bahmanyar S, Montgomery S. Multiple sclerosis and risk of attempted and completed suicide—a cohort study. *Eur J Neurol*. 2016;23(8):1329-1336.

128. Hardiman O, van den Berg LH, Kiernan MC. Clinical diagnosis and management of amyotrophic lateral sclerosis. *Nat Rev Neurol.* 2011;7(11):639-649.

129. Chio A, Logroscino G, Hardiman O, et al. Prognostic factors in ALS: A critical review. *Amyotroph Lateral Scler.* 2009;10(5-6):310-323.

130. Moura MC, Novaes MR, Eduardo EJ, Zago YS, Freitas Rdel N, Casulari LA. Prognostic factors in amyotrophic lateral sclerosis: a population-based study. *PLoS One.* 2015;10(10):e0141500.

131. Creemers H, Grupstra H, Nollet F, van den Berg LH, Beelen A. Prognostic factors for the course of functional status of patients with ALS: a systematic review. *J Neurol.* 2015;262(6):1407-1423.

132. Kappos L, Kuhle J, Multanen J, et al. Factors influencing long-term outcomes in relapsing-remitting multiple sclerosis: PRISMS-15. *J Neurol Neurosurg Psychiatry.* 2015;86(11):1202-1207.

133. Scott TF, Schramke CJ, Novero J, Chieffe C. Short-term prognosis in early relapsing-remitting multiple sclerosis. *Neurology.* 2000;55(5):689-693.

134. Bagert B, Camplair P, Bourdette D. Cognitive dysfunction in multiple sclerosis: natural history, pathophysiology and management. *CNS Drugs.* 2002;16(7):445-455.

135. Jauch EC, Saver JL, Adams HP, Jr., et al. Guidelines for the early management of patients with acute ischemic stroke: a guideline for healthcare professionals from the American Heart Association/American Stroke Association. *Stroke.* 2013;44(3):870-947.

136. Tsivgoulis G, Alleman J, Katsanos AH, et al. Comparative efficacy of different acute reperfusion therapies for acute ischemic stroke: a comprehensive benefit-risk analysis of clinical trials. *Brain Behav.* 2014;4(6):789-797.

137. Emberson J, Lees KR, Lyden P, et al. Effect of treatment delay, age, and stroke severity on the effects of intravenous thrombolysis with alteplase for acute ischaemic stroke: a meta-analysis of individual patient data from randomised trials. *Lancet.* 2014;384(9958):1929-1935.

138. Kate M, Gioia L, Buck B, et al. Dabigatran therapy in acute ischemic stroke patients without atrial fibrillation. *Stroke.* 2015;46(9):2685-2687.

139. Schiele F, van Ryn J, Canada K, et al. A specific antidote for dabigatran: functional and structural characterization. *Blood.* 2013;121(18):3554-3562.

140. Majeed A, Schulman S. Bleeding and antidotes in new oral anticoagulants. *Best Pract Res Clin Haematol.* 2013;26(2):191-202.

141. Hemphill JC, 3rd, Greenberg SM, Anderson CS, et al. Guidelines for the management of spontaneous intracerebral hemorrhage: a guideline for healthcare professionals from the American Heart Association/American Stroke Association. *Stroke.* 2015;46(7):2032-2060.

142. Bederson JB, Connolly ES, Jr., Batjer HH, et al. Guidelines for the management of aneurysmal subarachnoid hemorrhage: a statement for healthcare professionals from a special writing group of the Stroke Council, American Heart Association. *Stroke.* 2009;40(3):994-1025.

143. Berg A, Lonnqvist J, Palomaki H, Kaste M. Assessment of depression after stroke: a comparison of different screening instruments. *Stroke.* 2009;40(2):523-529.

144. Holloway RG, Arnold RM, Creutzfeldt CJ, et al. Palliative and end-of-life care in stroke: a statement for healthcare professionals from the American Heart Association/American Stroke Association. *Stroke.* 2014;45(6):1887-1916.

145. Nesbitt J, Moxham S, Ramadurai G, Williams L. Improving pain assessment and managment in stroke patients. *BMJ Qual Improv Rep.* 2015;4(1).

146. Schnakers C, Chatelle C, Majerus S, Gosseries O, De Val M, Laureys S. Assessment and detection of pain in noncommunicative severely brain-injured patients. *Expert Rev Neurother.* 2010;10(11):1725-1731.

147. Vestergaard K, Andersen G, Gottrup H, Kristensen BT, Jensen TS. Lamotrigine for central poststroke pain: a randomized controlled trial. *Neurology.* 2001;56(2):184-190.

148. Li Z, Alexander SA. Current evidence in the management of poststroke hemiplegic shoulder pain: a review. *J Neurosci Nurs.* 2015;47(1):10-19.

149. Francisco GE, McGuire JR. Poststroke spasticity management. *Stroke.* 2012;43(11):3132-3136.

150. Hubacher M, Calabrese P, Bassetti C, Carota A, Stocklin M, Penner IK. Assessment of post-stroke fatigue: the fatigue scale for motor and cognitive functions. *Eur Neurol.* 2012;67(6):377-384.

151. Mead G, Lynch J, Greig C, Young A, Lewis S, Sharpe M. Evaluation of fatigue scales in stroke patients. *Stroke.* 2007;38(7):2090-2095.

152. Brioschi A, Gramigna S, Werth E, et al. Effect of modafinil on subjective fatigue in multiple sclerosis and stroke patients. *Eur Neurol.* 2009;62(4):243-249.

153. Silverman IE, Restrepo L, Mathews GC. Poststroke seizures. *Arch Neurol.* 2002;59(2):195-201.

154. Fasano A, Daniele A, Albanese A. Treatment of motor and non-motor features of Parkinson's disease with deep brain stimulation. *Lancet Neurol.* 2012;11(5):429-442.

155. Kleiner-Fisman G, Herzog J, Fisman DN, et al. Subthalamic nucleus deep brain stimulation: summary and meta-analysis of outcomes. *Mov Disord.* 2006;21 Suppl 14:S290-304.

156. Voon V, Krack P, Lang AE, et al. A multicentre study on suicide outcomes following subthalamic stimulation for Parkinson's disease. *Brain.* 2008;131(Pt 10):2720-2728.

157. Miyasaki JM, Shannon K, Voon V, et al. Practice parameter: evaluation and treatment of depression, psychosis, and dementia in Parkinson disease (an evidence-based review): report of the Quality Standards Subcommittee of the American Academy of Neurology. *Neurology.* 2006;66(7):996-1002.

158. Bharucha KJ, Sethi KD. Complex movement disorders induced by fluoxetine. *Mov Disord.* 1996;11(3):324-326.

159. Richard IH, Kurlan R, Tanner C, et al. Serotonin syndrome and the combined use of deprenyl and an antidepressant in Parkinson's disease. Parkinson Study Group. *Neurology.* 1997;48(4):1070-1077.

160. Oliver D, Veronese S. Palliative approach to Parkinson disease and parkinsonian disorders. *UpToDate.* https://www.uptodate.com/contents/palliative-approach-to-parkinson-disease-and-parkinsonian-disorders. Accessed June 30, 2017.

161. Rana AQ, Kabir A, Jesudasan M, Siddiqui I, Khondker S. Pain in Parkinson's disease: analysis and literature review. *Clin Neurol Neurosurg.* 2013;115(11):2313-2317.

162. Ondo WG, Kenney C, Sullivan K, et al. Placebo-controlled trial of lubiprostone for constipation associated with Parkinson disease. *Neurology.* 2012;78(21):1650-1654.

163. Olek M. Disease-modifying treatment of relapsing-remitting multiple sclerosis in adults. *UpToDate.* https://www.uptodate.com/contents/disease-modifying-treatment-of-relapsing-remitting-multiple-sclerosis-in-adults. Accessed June 30, 2017.

164. Murray TJ. Diagnosis and treatment of multiple sclerosis. *BMJ.* 2006;332(7540):525-527.

165. Weinshenker BG. Plasma exchange for severe attacks of inflammatory demyelinating diseases of the central nervous system. *J Clin Apher.* 2001;16(1):39-42.

166. Attarian HP, Brown KM, Duntley SP, Carter JD, Cross AH. The relationship of sleep disturbances and fatigue in multiple sclerosis. *Arch Neurol.* 2004;61(4):525-528.

167. Tur C. Fatigue management in multiple sclerosis. *Curr Treat Options Neurol.* 2016;18(6):26.

168. Payne C, Wiffen PJ, Martin S. Interventions for fatigue and weight loss in adults with advanced progressive illness. *Cochrane Database Syst Rev.* 2012;1:Cd008427.

169. Taus C, Giuliani G, Pucci E, D'Amico R, Solari A. Amantadine for fatigue in multiple sclerosis. *Cochrane Database Syst Rev.* 2003(2):Cd002818.

170. Asano M, Finlayson ML. Meta-analysis of three different types of fatigue management interventions for people with multiple sclerosis: exercise, education, and medication. *Mult Scler Int.* 2014;2014:798285.

171. Wingerchuk DM, Benarroch EE, O'Brien PC, et al. A randomized controlled crossover trial of aspirin for fatigue in multiple sclerosis. *Neurology.* 2005;64(7):1267-1269.

172. Patten SB, Beck CA, Williams JV, Barbui C, Metz LM. Major depression in multiple sclerosis: a population-based perspective. *Neurology.* 2003;61(11):1524-1527.

173. Koch MW, Glazenborg A, Uyttenboogaart M, Mostert J, De Keyser J. Pharmacologic treatment of depression in multiple sclerosis. *Cochrane Database Syst Rev.* 2011(2):Cd007295.

174. Solaro C, Messmer Uccelli M. Pharmacological management of pain in patients with multiple sclerosis. *Drugs.* 2010;70(10):1245-1254.

175. Chou R, Peterson K, Helfand M. Comparative efficacy and safety of skeletal muscle relaxants for spasticity and musculoskeletal conditions: a systematic review. *J Pain Symptom Manage.* 2004;28(2):140-175.

176. Nyquist PA, Cascino GD, Rodriguez M. Seizures in patients with multiple sclerosis seen at Mayo Clinic, Rochester, Minn, 1990-1998. *Mayo Clin Proc.* 2001;76(10):983-986.

177. Chiaravalloti ND, DeLuca J. Cognitive impairment in multiple sclerosis. *Lancet Neurol.* 2008;7(12):1139-1151.

178. Goodman AD, Brown TR, Krupp LB, et al. Sustained-release oral fampridine in multiple sclerosis: a randomised, double-blind, controlled trial. *Lancet.* 2009;373(9665):732-738.

179. Bensimon G, Lacomblez L, Meininger V. A controlled trial of riluzole in amyotrophic lateral sclerosis. ALS/Riluzole Study Group. *N Engl J Med.* 1994;330(9):585-591.

180. Lacomblez L, Bensimon G, Leigh PN, Guillet P, Meininger V. Dose-ranging study of riluzole in amyotrophic lateral sclerosis. Amyotrophic Lateral Sclerosis/Riluzole Study Group II. *Lancet.* 1996;347(9013):1425-1431.

181. Miller RG, Mitchell JD, Moore DH. Riluzole for amyotrophic lateral sclerosis (ALS)/motor neuron disease (MND). *Cochrane Database Syst Rev.* 2012;3:Cd001447.

182. Galvez-Jimenez N. Symptom-based management of amyotrophic lateral sclerosis. *UpToDate.* https://www.uptodate.com/contents/symptom-based-management-of-amyotrophic-lateral-sclerosis. Accessed June 30, 2017.

183. Miller RG, Jackson CE, Kasarskis EJ, et al. Practice parameter update: the care of the patient with amyotrophic lateral sclerosis: drug, nutritional, and respiratory therapies (an evidence-based review): report of the Quality Standards Subcommittee of the American Academy of Neurology. *Neurology.* 2009;73(15):1218-1226.

184. Ahmed A, Simmons Z. Pseudobulbar affect: prevalence and management. *Ther Clin Risk Manag.* 2013;9:483-489.

185. Rabkin JG, Gordon PH, McElhiney M, Rabkin R, Chew S, Mitsumoto H. Modafinil treatment of fatigue in patients with ALS: a placebo-controlled study. *Muscle Nerve.* 2009;39(3):297-303.

186. Borasio GD, Voltz R, Miller RG. Palliative care in amyotrophic lateral sclerosis. *Neurol Clin.* 2001;19(4):829-847.

187. Katzberg HD, Benatar M. Enteral tube feeding for amyotrophic lateral sclerosis/motor neuron disease. *Cochrane Database Syst Rev.* 2011(1):Cd004030.

188. Diener BL, Bischof-Rosarioz JA. Determining decision-making capacity in individuals with severe communication impairments after stroke: the role of augmentative-alternative communication (AAC). *Top Stroke Rehabil.* 2004;11(1):84-88.

189. Singh S, Hamdy S. Dysphagia in stroke patients. *Postgrad Med J.* 2006;82(968):383-391.

190. Poorjavad M, Derakhshandeh F, Etemadifar M, Soleymani B, Minagar A, Maghzi AH. Oropharyngeal dysphagia in multiple sclerosis. *Mult Scler.* 2010;16(3):362-365.

191. Higginson IJ, Gao W, Saleem TZ, et al. Symptoms and quality of life in late stage Parkinson syndromes: a longitudinal community study of predictive factors. *PLoS One.* 2012;7(11):e46327.

192. Cucca A, Mazzucco S, Bursomanno A, et al. Amino acid supplementation in l-dopa treated Parkinson's disease patients. *Clin Nutr.* 2015;34(6):1189-1194.

193. Plonk W. To PEG or not to PEG. *Pract Gastroenterol.* 2005;24(7):16, 19-26, 31. www.practicalgastro.com/pdf/July05/July05Plonk.pdf. Accessed June 30, 2017.

194. Maltoni M, Scarpi E, Rosati M, et al. Palliative sedation in end-of-life care and survival: a systematic review. *J Clin Oncol.* 2012;30(12):1378-1383.

195. Miyasaki JM, Long J, Mancini D, et al. Palliative care for advanced Parkinson disease: an interdisciplinary clinic and new scale, the ESAS-PD. *Parkinsonism Relat Disord.* 2012;18 Suppl 3:S6-9.

196. Kim Y, Schulz R. Family caregivers' strains: comparative analysis of cancer caregiving with dementia, diabetes, and frail elderly caregiving. *J Aging Health.* 2008;20(5):483-503.

197. Clarke DM, McLeod JE, Smith GC, Trauer T, Kissane DW. A comparison of psychosocial and physical functioning in patients with motor neurone disease and metastatic cancer. *J Palliat Care.* 2005;21(3):173-179.

198. Teno JM, Clarridge BR, Casey V, et al. Family perspectives on end-of-life care at the last place of care. *JAMA.* 2004;291(1):88-93.

199. Thorpe KE, Howard DH. The rise in spending among Medicare beneficiaries: the role of chronic disease prevalence and changes in treatment intensity. *Health Aff (Millwood).* 2006;25(5):w378-388.

200. Meier DE. Increased access to palliative care and hospice services: opportunities to improve value in health care. *Milbank Q.* 2011;89(3):343-380.

201. National Hospice and Palliative Care Organization. NHPCO's Facts and Figures: Hospice Care in America. 2015 ed. Arlington, VA: National Hospice and Palliative Care Organization. www.nhpco.org/sites/default/files/public/Statistics_Research/2015_Facts_Figures.pdf. Accessed June 30, 2017.

202. Sleeman KE, Ho YK, Verne J, et al. Place of death, and its relation with underlying cause of death, in Parkinson's disease, motor neuron disease, and multiple sclerosis: a population-based study. *Palliat Med.* 2013;27(9):840-846.

203. Corcia P, Pradat PF, Salachas F, et al. Causes of death in a post-mortem series of ALS patients. *Amyotroph Lateral Scler.* 2008;9(1):59-62.

204. Vernino S, Brown RD, Jr., Sejvar JJ, Sicks JD, Petty GW, O'Fallon WM. Cause-specific mortality after first cerebral infarction: a population-based study. *Stroke.* 2003;34(8):1828-1832.

205. Capkun G, Dahlke F, Lahoz R, et al. Mortality and comorbidities in patients with multiple sclerosis compared with a population without multiple sclerosis: An observational study using the US Department of Defense administrative claims database. *Mult Scler Relat Disord.* 2015;4(6):546-554.

206. Centers for Medicare and Medicaid Services, US Department of Health and Human Services. Local Coverage Determinations (LCDs) by Contractor Index. www.cms.gov/medicare-coverage-database/indexes/lcd-contractor-index.aspx. Accessed June 27, 2017.

207. Martinez-Martin P, Forjaz MJ, Frades-Payo B, et al. Caregiver burden in Parkinson's disease. *Mov Disord.* 2007;22(7):924-931; quiz 1060.

208. Burke T, Elamin M, Galvin M, Hardiman O, Pender N. Caregiver burden in amyotrophic lateral sclerosis: a cross-sectional investigation of predictors. *J Neurol.* 2015;262(6):1526-1532.

209. Buchanan RJ, Radin D, Huang C. Caregiver burden among informal caregivers assisting people with multiple sclerosis. *Int J MS Care.* 2011;13(2):76-83.

210. van Exel NJ, Koopmanschap MA, van den Berg B, Brouwer WB, van den Bos GA. Burden of informal caregiving for stroke patients. Identification of caregivers at risk of adverse health effects. *Cerebrovasc Dis.* 2005;19(1):11-17.

211. Bock M, Duong YN, Kim A, Allen I, Murphy J, Lomen-Hoerth C. Cognitive-behavioral changes in amyotrophic lateral sclerosis: Screening prevalence and impact on patients and caregivers. *Amyotroph Lateral Scler Frontotemporal Degener.* 2016;17(5-6):366-373.

212. McCullagh E, Brigstocke G, Donaldson N, Kalra L. Determinants of caregiving burden and quality of life in caregivers of stroke patients. *Stroke.* 2005;36(10):2181-2186.

213. Adelman RD, Tmanova LL, Delgado D, Dion S, Lachs MS. Caregiver burden: a clinical review. *JAMA.* 2014;311(10):1052-1060.

214. Cochrane JJ, Goering PN, Rogers JM. The mental health of informal caregivers in Ontario: an epidemiological survey. *Am J Public Health.* 1997;87(12):2002-2007.

215. Schulz R, Beach SR. Caregiving as a risk factor for mortality: the Caregiver Health Effects Study. *JAMA.* 1999;282(23):2215-2219.

216. Rodakowski J, Skidmore ER, Rogers JC, Schulz R. Role of social support in predicting caregiver burden. *Arch Phys Med Rehabil.* 2012;93(12):2229-2236.

217. Zarit SH, Reever KE, Bach-Peterson J. Relatives of the impaired elderly: correlates of feelings of burden. *Gerontologist.* 1980;20(6):649-655.

# Index